The COVID-19 Pandemic in the Middle East and North Africa

W0113041

This book critically reflects on the responses to the COVID-19 pandemic in the Middle East and North Africa (MENA) by exploring the impact and possible future outcomes in a region already struggling with the effects of a decade of uprisings, failed or difficult political transitions, state collapses, civil war, and international conflict. International scholars offer a comprehensive treatment of today's major societal issues and provide a unique, broadly comparative view on public policy responses in the MENA region. Addressing the implications and public policy responses to the crisis, they bring a critical perspective to the emerging challenges of evidence-based policy making; the locus of authority in transnational issues; the nature of governance; and the role of government and implications for civil society. Tackling the psychology, sociology, education, law, and public policy issues related to the social and economic implications of the COVID-19 pandemic, this book will be of interest to scholars and students alike.

Dr Anis Ben Brik is an associate professor and founding director of the Program for Social Policy Evaluation and Research (PROSPER) at the College of Public Policy, Hamad Bin Khalifa University (HBKU). Before joining HBKU, Dr Ben Brik served as director of the Family Policy Department at the Doha International Family Institute. He previously served as a senior policy advisor and consultant to many government ministries and organizations in the Middle East and North Africa region.

The Politics of Pandemics

Understanding the Politics of Pandemic Emergencies in the time of COVID-19
An Introduction to Global Politosomatics
Mika Aaltola

Pandemic Response and the Cost of Lockdowns
Global Debates from Humanities and Social Sciences
Edited by Peter Sutoris, Sinéad Murphy, Aleida Mendes Borges and Yossi Nehushtan

The COVID-19 Pandemic in the Middle East and North Africa
Public Policy Responses
Edited by Anis Ben Brik

For more information see https://www.routledge.com/The-Politics-of-Pandemics/book-series/TPOP

The COVID-19 Pandemic in the Middle East and North Africa

Public Policy Responses

Edited by
Anis Ben Brik

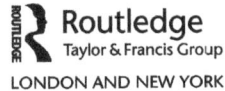
Routledge
Taylor & Francis Group

LONDON AND NEW YORK

First published 2023
by Routledge
4 Park Square, Milton Park, Abingdon, Oxon OX14 4RN

and by Routledge
605 Third Avenue, New York, NY 10158

Routledge is an imprint of the Taylor & Francis Group, an informa business

© 2023 selection and editorial matter, Anis Ben Brik; individual chapters, the contributors

The right of Anis Ben Brik to be identified as the author of the editorial material, and of the authors for their individual chapters, has been asserted in accordance with sections 77 and 78 of the Copyright, Designs and Patents Act 1988.

All rights reserved. No part of this book may be reprinted or reproduced or utilised in any form or by any electronic, mechanical, or other means, now known or hereafter invented, including photocopying and recording, or in any information storage or retrieval system, without permission in writing from the publishers.

Trademark notice: Product or corporate names may be trademarks or registered trademarks, and are used only for identification and explanation without intent to infringe.

British Library Cataloguing-in-Publication Data
A catalogue record for this book is available from the British Library

Library of Congress Cataloging-in-Publication Data
Names: Brik, Anis Ben, editor.
Title: The COVID-19 pandemic in the Middle East and North Africa : public policy responses / edited by Anis Ben Brik.
Description: Abingdon, Oxon ; New York, NY : Routledge, 2023. | Series: The politics of pandemics | Includes bibliographical references and index.
Identifiers: LCCN 2022014130 (print) | LCCN 2022014131 (ebook) | ISBN 9781032209661 (hardback) | ISBN 9781032209913 (paperback) | ISBN 9781003266259 (ebook)
Subjects: LCSH: COVID-19 Pandemic, 2020—Middle East. | COVID-19 Pandemic, 2020—Africa, North. | COVID-19 (Disease)—Government policy—Middle East. | COVID-19 (Disease)—Government policy—Africa, North.
Classification: LCC RA644.C67 C6827 2022 (print) | LCC RA644. C67 (ebook) | DDC 362.1962/414—dc23/eng/20220520
LC record available at https://lccn.loc.gov/2022014130
LC ebook record available at https://lccn.loc.gov/2022014131

ISBN: 978-1-032-20966-1 (hbk)
ISBN: 978-1-032-20991-3 (pbk)
ISBN: 978-1-003-26625-9 (ebk)

DOI: 10.4324/9781003266259

Typeset in Times New Roman
by codeMantra

Contents

Figures

Tables

Contributors

Hamid Ait El Caid is a PhD student in Political Science and International Relations at Corvinus University of Budapest, Hungary.

Lucia Ardovini is a lecturer in International Relations in the Department of Politics, Philosophy and Religion at Lancaster University, UK and author of *Surviving Repression: the Egyptian Muslim Brotherhood after the 2013 coup* (2022).

Anis Ben Brik is an associate professor at Hamad Bin Khalifa University, College of Public Policy, Qatar and co-author of *The Future of the Policy Sciences* (2021).

Abdelhakim Aboullouz is an assistant professor at the University Ibn Zohr, Morocco

Nejla Ben Mimoune is a research assistant at the Brookings Doha Center, Qatar.

Diana Galeeva is an academic visitor to St. Antony's College, University of Oxford, UK and author of *Qatar: The Practice of Rented Power* (Routledge, 2022).

Ali Maleki is a researcher at Sharif Policy Research Institute (SPRI), Sharif University of Technology, Iran.

Alhafad Nouini is a researcher in Political Science and International Law at the Universidad de Santiago de Compostela, Spain.

Ozcan Ozturk is an assistant professor at Hamad Bin Khalifa University, College of Public Policy, Qatar.

Leslie A. Pal is the founding dean of the College of Public Policy at Hamad Bin Khalifa University, Qatar and co-author of *The Future of the Policy Sciences* (2021).

Andreas Rechkemmer is a professor at Hamad Bin Khalifa University, College of Public Policy, Qatar and co-author of the *Oxford Handbook of Complex Disaster Risks and Resilience* (2020).

Najmoddin Yazdi is a researcher at Sharif Policy Research Institute (SPRI), Sharif University of Technology, Iran.

1 Introduction

Facing the Wave: A Journey in the Shadow of the Pandemic

Anis Ben Brik

The Middle East in the Shadow of the Pandemic

The Middle East and North Africa (MENA) region comprises a mix of high-income countries (Bahrain, Kuwait, Oman, Qatar, Saudi Arabia, and the UAE); upper-middle-income countries (Iran, Iraq, Jordan, Lebanon, and Libya); some lower-middle-income countries and economies (Algeria, the Arab Republic of Egypt, Morocco, Tunisia, and Palestine); and some low-income countries (Algeria, the Arab Republic of Egypt, Syria, and Yemen). Additionally, while some countries are heavily reliant on oil exports (Algeria, Gulf Cooperation Council countries, and the Islamic Republic of Iran), others are either mired in a pre-existing financial crisis (the Islamic Republic of Iran and Lebanon) or are experiencing protests and social unrest (Algeria, Lebanon, and Tunisia). Additionally, some are characterized by fragility, conflict, and violence-related vulnerabilities, including (a) high-intensity conflict in Libya and Syria, (b) medium-intensity conflict in Iraq and Yemen, (c) social fragility in Lebanon and Palestine, and (d) spillover effects in Jordan and Lebanon. Additionally, the region continues to face climate risks, including water scarcity, coastal flooding, desertification, and famine (Hoogeveen and Lopez-Acevedo, 2021).

The coronavirus pandemic has swept through a region already struggling to recover from the effects of a decade of uprisings, failed or stalled political transitions, state fragility and failure, economic decline, collapsing social safety nets, civil war, and international conflict. For example, the region has recently seen a new wave of "Arab Uprisings" against regimes that have exacerbated inequalities and social vulnerabilities. People in Sudan, Algeria, Lebanon, and Iraq demonstrated against skyrocketing living costs, deteriorating living conditions, rising rates of unemployment and poverty, the inaccessibility of a privatized healthcare system, the continuation of violence against women, the "corruption" of ruling elites, and the inability of current governments to provide a minimum level of social protection.

The majority of MENA countries have struggled to provide adequate health care and social assistance to their most vulnerable citizens. Conflict-affected MENA countries, as well as fragile states such as Iraq,

DOI: 10.4324/9781003266259-1

Somalia, Sudan, and Palestine, are in a particularly precarious position. Other MENA countries, including Lebanon, Iran, and Tunisia, are grappling with political crises or financial constraints that impair their ability to provide critical public services. Numerous states also have refugee populations that face coverage gaps. Even stable countries like Egypt, Jordan, Morocco, and Algeria struggle to meet basic social needs. Additionally, the pandemic exposed and amplified these institutional weaknesses throughout the region. Indeed, the pandemic serves as a unique "stress test" for the various institutional conditions and governance constraints prevalent in MENA countries. It provides an opportunity to investigate institutional responses and coping mechanisms that could assist policymakers in improving service delivery. Additionally, it enables policymakers and the international community to assess which capacity gaps are truly structural and which can be addressed through a combination of technical assistance and political will.

The global COVID-19 pandemic is wreaking havoc on welfare systems, institutions, and society throughout the region, with far-reaching social consequences. Additionally, the COVID-19 crisis generates considerable concern among policymakers and researchers. Measures taken across the region to halt the virus's spread, such as the suspension of schools and universities, have disrupted a generation of students' learning and lives. Additionally, the closures disproportionately affect disadvantaged women, children, and adolescents, who have fewer educational opportunities outside of school and limited access to remote learning tools and the Internet. They frequently also rely on free or reduced school meals to maintain healthy nutrition. The coronavirus pandemic has been particularly hard on the region in this context.

Many governments throughout the region are now under increased pressure to enhance the quality of public services. For example, the enduring effects of the youth bulge have distinct implications for labor markets and housing demand, putting enormous strain on the region's already overburdened social policy regimes. In many countries, refugee flows impose enormous strains on social sectors and government capacities to meet the demands of citizens and non-citizens alike. These changes have imposed fundamental questions on policymakers and researchers, who are being pressed to reconsider conventional public policy approaches. Additionally, national governments' ability to combat the pandemic and its economic and social consequences is contingent upon political factors and national institutions. Welfare state institutions and social policies, in particular, face significant challenges in ensuring social security and stabilizing the economy. The COVID-19 pandemic has had a significant impact on the responsibilities of welfare state organizations in terms of ensuring rapid access to welfare payments and providing extensive job security. Additionally, the pandemic may alter the objectives, design, and implementation of social and labor market policies. Additionally, it has consequences for public services.

The book provides a comprehensive assessment of the pandemic's implications and generates new and cutting-edge knowledge about this novel global threat, as well as its implications for the MENA region. The book examines the social and economic implications of the COVID-19 pandemic, social cohesion, freedom of expression, vulnerable populations, resilience, authoritarianism, and institutional reforms from the perspectives of psychology, sociology, education, law, and public policy. The book provides a critical analysis of the emerging challenges confronting MENA societies in the aftermath of the pandemic and initiates dialogue among scholars from diverse disciplines.

The book addresses several significant knowledge gaps regarding the pandemic's implications and public policy responses in the MENA region. It examines the following questions: what are the pandemic's social, economic, and political consequences?; how have MENA countries responded to the pandemic?; what are the key factors underlying the region's diversity of national responses to the pandemic?; how does the response to the pandemic affect the region's struggle for freedom of expression and social justice?; how might the pandemic restructure, reshape, or challenge social policies or welfare regimes in the Gulf region?; what gaps in service delivery and institutional capacities have been exposed?; what inequalities are being highlighted by the pandemic and policy responses?; what are the implications of the pandemic on vulnerable populations?; how does the pandemic impact job security or unemployment?; what is the role of social protection in mitigating the impacts of COVID-19?; what will the region look like after the pandemic?; what are the prospects for improved governance?; what steps should governments take today to ensure that lessons translate into better policies?; and which welfare state models are more resilient to retrenchment and why?

The book brings a critical perspective to the emerging challenges of evidence-based policymaking; implications of the pandemic for the locus of authority in terms of the rise of transnational issues; implications for the nature of governance and the role of government; and implications for civil-society, representation, and political contestation. Overall, the book is a critical stocktaking and reflection on the implications and public policy responses, its strengths and weaknesses, and where it may or should be heading in the future as well as open lines of inquiry among scholars from diverse disciplines.

Epidemiological Situation, Health Preparedness, and Systems

On January 29, 2020, the UAE reported the first coronavirus case in the MENA region. The disease then spread from east to west, with Egypt reporting the second positive case on February 15, followed by the remaining countries in the region, which all reported cases within the next 15 days (except countries in conflict, which reported reporting cases in mid-March, with Yemen reporting the final positive case on April 11) (UNDP, 2020).

By the end of January 2022, the MENA region would have accumulated over 13 million confirmed COVID cases and over 244,000 confirmed COVID-19 deaths (World Bank, 2021a). According to official statistics, COVID-19 has surpassed malaria as the region's fifth leading cause of death (assuming causes of death in 2020 were otherwise comparable to 2019). However, factors such as test positivity rates, seroprevalence (the actual infection rate), and well-documented widespread disruptions of health services suggest that the impact of COVID-19 is grossly underestimated. The number of reported COVID-19 cases per million population, the total number of cases and deaths, and the number of deaths per million population are shown in Table 1.1. Bahrain (252,615), Lebanon (148,479), Jordan (138,595), and Kuwait (136,487) have the highest case fatality rate per million. Tunisia (2,247) has the region's highest death rate per 100,000, followed by Iran (1,557) and Lebanon (1,447) (Worldometer, 2022).

Health Preparedness

Prior to the onset of COVID-19, health inequality was widespread in the MENA region and closely mirrored income disparities, which are particularly pronounced in this region due to its diverse development profiles.

Table 1.1 Total cases per million population and fatality rate as of January 31, 2021

	Testing/1 million	Total testing	Vaccination rates: % of country population vaccinated
Tunisia	349,357	4,198,650	52
Iran	530,818	45,505,835	64
Lebanon	707,720	4,795,578	30
Jordan	1,493,252	15,479,967	41
Palestine	581,663	3,078,533	30
Libya	331,648	2,328,851	14
Bahrain	5,083,722	9,134,783	68
Oman	1,060,646	20,184,607	57
Iraq	424,888	17,708,484	15
Kuwait	1,664,839	7,279,468	75
Morocco	298,725	11,237,010	62
Saudi Arabia	1,104,011	39,400,621	67
Qatar	1,189,373	3,339,527	77
UAE	13,000,417	131,086,391	93
Egypt	35,026	3,693,367	26
Syria	8,043	146,269	6
Algeria	5,116	230,861	14
Yemen	8,588	265,253	1
Sudan	12,372	562,941	4
Mauritania	147,583	715,290	20
MENA region	28,037,807	320,372,286	

Source: Worldometer (https://www.worldometers.info/coronavirus/).

Inequalities in life expectancy and health outcomes are evident and persistent, both between and within the region's countries, not least because the region contains eight of the world's 36 most fragile and crisis-prone countries (World Bank, 2021b).

As illustrated in Table 1.2, the pandemic exposed fundamental shortcomings in health preparedness: health expenditure as a percentage of GDP and hospital beds per 10,000 people. For example, oil-exporting countries lead the region in terms of health infrastructure and human resources for health – according to the most recent available data, Kuwait has the highest ratio of medical doctors per 10,000 population – 26.5 – and 74.2 nurses and midwives per 10,000 population – while Bahrain has the lowest ratio of medical doctors per 10,000 population – 9.3 – and Algeria has the lowest ratio of nurses per 10,000 population – 15.5 – (WHO, 2021a). Additionally, oil-importing, middle-income countries have lower levels of preparedness and infrastructure, with medical doctor availability ranging from 2.2 (Djibouti) to 23.2 (Jordan) and nurse availability ranging from 7.3 (Djibouti) to 28.2 (Jordan) (Jordan). Fragile countries have extremely underdeveloped health systems, with physician availability ranging from 0.2 (Somalia) to 21 (Lebanon) and nurse availability ranging from 1.1 (Somalia) to 65.3 (Libya) (WHO, 2021b).

Table 1.2 Health preparedness in MENA countries

	GDP, current prices (billions of U.S. dollars), 2021–2022	Human development index (HDI)	Inequality in HDI	Hospital beds (per 10,000 population)	Medical doctors (per 10,000 population)	Nurses and midwifes (per 10,000 population)
Tunisia	45.4	0.739	20.8	21.8	13	25.1
Lebanon	21.8	0.73	n.a	27.3	20.9	65.3
Jordan	47.5	0.723	14.7	14.7	23.2	28.2
Palestine	18.78	0.69	13.5	n.a	n.a	n.a
Libya	29.2	0.708	n.a	32	20.9	65.3
Bahrain	41.06	0.838	n.a	17.4	9.3	24.9
Oman	85.72	0.834	12.2	14.7	20	42
Iraq	226.62	0.689	19.8	13.2	7.1	20.5
Kuwait	138.78	0.808	n.a	20.4	26.5	74.2
Morocco	132.65	0.676	n.a	10	7.3	13.9
Saudi Arabia	876.15	0.857	n.a	22.4	26.1	54.8
Qatar	180.88	0.848	n.a	12.5	24.9	72.6
UAE	427.93	0.866	n.a	13.8	25.3	57.3
Egypt	438.35	0.7	29.7	14.3	4.5	19.3
Syria	27.26	0.549	n.a	14	12.9	15.4
Algeria	168.2	0.759	20.4	19	17.2	15.5
Yemen	20.02	0.463	31.8	7.1	5.3	7.9
Sudan	37.77	0.507	34.6	7.4	2.6	7
Djibouti	3.93	0.495	n.a	14	2.2	7.3
World		0.731	18.6	28	15.6	37.6

Sources: United Nations Development Programme (UNDP).
Note: n.a: data not available.

COVID-19 Testing and Vaccinations

COVID-19 vaccine distribution is significantly unequal throughout the region, with the vast majority of doses acquired and administered in the region's wealthiest countries. As of January 31, 2022, Table 1.3 shows the number of tests performed per million population and vaccination rates for each country. The Arabian Gulf countries, specifically the UAE (13,000,417), Bahrain (5,083,722), and Qatar (1,189,373), lead the region in terms of tests per million (Worldometer, 2022). Algeria (5,116), Syria (8,043), and Yemen (8,588) have the region's lowest testing rates. The data demonstrate significant disparities in coronavirus testing across MENA countries. Additionally, vaccine inequality is becoming more pronounced throughout the region. While the UAE, Qatar, and Kuwait lead the region in terms of fully vaccinated populations at 93%, 77%, and 75%, respectively, Syria, Yemen, and Sudan have less than 5% fully vaccinated populations.

Healthcare Systems

The pandemic struck the majority of MENA countries, which had underfunded, inefficient, and unprepared healthcare systems (Gatti et al., 2021). COVID-19 imposed severe demands on MENA health systems, which already struggled to cope with truncated economic, demographic, and epidemiological transitions. On the eve of the pandemic, the capacity of MENA's public health systems to deploy resources and deliver both individual health care and critical public health functions was emphasized (World Bank, 2021b). The MENA region lacked a plethora of basic tools necessary for health service delivery, including essential medicines. COVID-19 exacerbated the strain on MENA's health systems by increasing demand for critical medical supplies such as oxygen, COVID-19 vaccines, and ventilators.

The 2019 Global Health Security Index, a ranking of 195 countries, provides a complementary perspective on relative national health sector capabilities. This includes health system criteria – health capacity in clinics, hospitals, and community healthcare centers; supply chain for health systems and healthcare workers; healthcare access; communication with healthcare workers during a public health emergency; infection control practices; and capacity to test and approve countermeasures (GHSI, 2019). None of the MENA countries are ranked among the world's top 50. The Arab Gulf states and Jordan are considered to be among the "more prepared" countries (Table 1.4).

Healthcare Spending

MENA countries face significant, albeit distinct, funding challenges for their health systems. In MENA countries, the average healthcare expenditure as a percentage of GDP is 5.96%, which is lower than in other regions. North America accounts for 16.42% of GDP, the OECD accounts for

Table 1.3 COVID-19 tests per million of population and vaccination rate as of January 31, 2021

	Testing/1 million	*Total testing*	*Vaccination rates: % of country population vaccinated*
Tunisia	349,357	4,198,650	52
Iran	530,818	45,505,835	64
Lebanon	707,720	4,795,578	30
Jordan	1,493,252	15,479,967	41
Palestine	581,663	3,078,533	30
Libya	331,648	2,328,851	14
Bahrain	5,083,722	9,134,783	68
Oman	1,060,646	20,184,607	57
Iraq	424,888	17,708,484	15
Kuwait	1,664,839	7,279,468	75
Morocco	298,725	11,237,010	62
Saudi Arabia	1,104,011	39,400,621	67
Qatar	1,189,373	3,339,527	77
UAE	13,000,417	131,086,391	93
Egypt	35,026	3,693,367	26
Syria	8,043	146,269	5
Algeria	5,116	230,861	14
Yemen	8,588	265,253	1
Sudan	12,372	562,941	4
Mauritania	147,583	715,290	20

Source: Worldometer (https://www.worldometers.info/coronavirus/).

Table 1.4 Multidimensional poverty measures in selected MENA countries

	Multidimensional poverty index	*Population in severe multidimensional poverty (%)*	*Population vulnerable to multidimensional poverty (%)*	*National poverty line (2009–2019)*	*PPP $1. 90 a day (2009–2019)*
Tunisia (2018)	0.8	0.1	2.4	15.2	0.2
Jordan (2017–2018)	0.4	0	0.7	14.4	0.1
Palestine (2019/2020)	0.002	0	1.3	29.2	0.8
Libya (2014)	2	0.1	11.4	n.a	n.a
Iraq (2018)	8.6	1.3	5.2	18.9	2.5
Morocco (2017/2018)	0.027	1.4	10.9	4.8	0.9
Egypt (2014)	5.2	0.6	6.1	32.5	3.2
Syria (2009)	7.4	1.2	7.8	n.a	n.a
Algeria (2018–2019)	0.005	0.2	3.6	5.5	0.4
Yemen (2013)	47.7	23.9	22.1	48.6	18.8
Sudan	52.3	30.9	17.7	46.5	12.7

Source: The 2021 Global Multidimensional Poverty Index, UNDP and OPHI (2021).

12.46%, Europe accounts for 10.14%, and East Asia and the Pacific accounts for 6.67% (Balkhi et al., 2021). Lebanon, Tunisia, and Saudi Arabia spend 8.35%, 7.29%, and 6.36% of GDP on health, respectively, which is higher than the UAE (3.3%), Kuwait (2.7%), Oman (2.3%), and Qatar (2.49%) (Table 1.5) (UNDP and OPHI, 2021).

Additionally, the regional Atlas of Health Financing indicated that between 2000 and 2015, the share of out-of-pocket (OOP) payments in the region fluctuated around 40% of the total current health expenditure, compared to a global average of 32% in 2015 (WHO, 2021b).

Gatti et al. (2021) demonstrate that on the eve of the pandemic, MENA's public health authorities painted rosy pictures of their public healthcare systems. Their self-reported indicators of preparedness were consistently more optimistic than those of comparable-development countries, while objective indicators showed MENA countries underperforming their peers, with Jordan being a notable exception.

In summary, COVID-19 exposed the majority of MENA countries' underfunded, unbalanced, and unprepared healthcare systems, further depleting limited functional and reserve capacities, exacerbating existing challenges, and exposing vulnerabilities that could no longer be compensated for. Thus, the pandemic served as a stress test for the healthcare system's resilience, emphasizing the critical nature of meeting previously unmet healthcare needs (Gatti et al., 2021).

Pandemic Economic Impacts

The MENA region has long faced structural challenges, including low GDP growth; low employment, particularly among youth and women; a low

Table 1.5 Health expenditure (CHE) (percentage of GDP), 2009–2019

	2009	2010	2011	2012	2013	2014	2015	2016	2017	2018	2019	*Average*
Tunisia	5.67	5.88	6.43	6.61	6.86	6.81	6.62	6.61	6.85	6.82	6.96	6.56
Lebanon	7.01	7.44	8.18	7	7.06	7.52	7.41	7.91	7.79	8.67	8.65	7.69
Jordan	9.22	8.17	8.15	7.82	7.17	7.21	7.46	7.16	7.98	7.78	7.58	7.79
Bahrain	4.06	3.84	3.58	4.11	4.31	4.41	4.99	4.86	4.74	4.14	4.01	4.28
Oman	2.83	2.82	2.55	2.55	2.79	3.53	4.3	4.36	3.97	4.1	4.07	3.44
Iran	6.5	6.69	6.57	6.58	5.94	6.76	7.54	8.57	8.43	8.46	6.71	7.16
Iraq	3.77	3.23	2.79	2.69	2.82	2.8	3.14	3.49	4.19	4.24	4.48	3.42
Kuwait	2.71	2.68	2.33	2.33	2.49	2.92	4.21	4.73	4.65	5.1	5.5	3.60
Morocco	5.84	5.86	5.73	5.75	5.69	5.28	5.07	5.24	5.23	5.33	5.31	5.48
Saudi Arabia	4.29	3.65	3.71	4.02	4.47	5.23	6	5.84	6.26	5.75	5.69	4.99
Qatar	2.38	1.87	1.6	1.75	2.08	2.42	3	3.25	2.98	2.63	2.91	2.44
UAE	4.05	3.88	3.67	3.43	3.59	3.63	3.58	3.47	4.06	4.15	4.28	3.80
Egypt	4.38	4.15	4.36	4.71	4.92	5.03	5.34	5.36	5.63	4.95	4.74	4.87
Algeria	5.36	5.12	5.27	6	6.04	6.55	6.98	6.61	6.28	6.16	6.24	6.06
Sudan	6.39	5.06	5.62	5.69	6.96	5.68	7.27	5.48	6.06	4.44	4.57	5.75
Djibouti	3.21	3.06	3.38	3.3	2.92	2.97	3.08	2.73	2.46	2.26	1.8	2.83

Source: WHO, Global Health Observatory data repository.

human capital index; a large informal sector; insufficient foreign direct investment inflows; a weak investment climate; insufficient participation in global value chains; and rising debt levels. These pre-existing conditions, which reflect the precarious state of the social contract in many countries throughout the region, have exacerbated the negative effects of COVID-19 (Hoogeveen and Lopez-Acevedo, 2021). MENA has experienced a low annual growth rate of about 1.4% per capita over the last two decades, significantly lower than its peers. Extreme poverty has more than doubled, from 2.4% in 2011 to 4.2% in 2015, owing in part to the conflicts in Libya, Syria, and Yemen. Even food insecurity has increased in recent years.

Lockdown measures, workplace closures, disrupted supply chains, dramatic declines in tourism and labor remittances, and temporarily low oil prices have stifled economic activity and widened inequalities by disproportionately affecting the poorest households, which are largely employed in informal sectors, lack health insurance, and are more susceptible to infection as a result of cramped living conditions across the region. For example, as oil prices fell, oil-exporting economies felt the brunt of the fiscal ripple effect, which resulted in lower private consumption and reduced energy sector investment. GDP contraction also occurs in oil-importing economies as investments dwindle and private consumption, a significant driver of GDP, declines. Many MENA countries' already high unemployment rates will continue to rise, especially among youth and women. Additionally, the tourism sector, which accounts for up to 20% of GDP in some MENA countries, has been decimated by the pandemic, with countries sealing off historic sites and closing their borders to visitors. The transportation sector is suffering, particularly Gulf airlines, many of which serve as major transit hubs. International trade has weakened, affecting the logistics industry and threatening to disrupt industries such as automobile manufacturing in Morocco and Tunisia, as well as textile manufacturing in Jordan. Finally, the wholesale, retail, and construction sectors in the region are all at risk of declining consumer demand.

Prior to the lockdown, the region's per capita GDP was estimated to be around US$14,000, then fell to slightly more than US$13,000 in 2020, and is expected to remain below US$14,000 until 2024 or 2025. Furthermore, it is estimated that MENA's output fell by more than 5% in 2020, with recovery unlikely until 2024 or 2025. Meanwhile, the economic cost of the pandemic in the region is estimated to be approximately US$227 billion (World Bank, 2021b), and fiscal support packages average 2.7% of GDP, further straining MENA's already precarious fiscal position.

Additionally, MENA is the only region in which poverty levels have been increasing since 2013. In countries such as Algeria (2018–2019), Egypt (2014), Jordan (2017–2018), and Tunisia (2018), less than 6% of the population is classified as multidimensional poor, whereas in Sudan (2014) and Yemen (2013), more than 40% of the population is classified as multidimensionally poor (Table 1.6). The MENA region has seen a significant increase in poverty rates as a result of COVID-19. According to a January World Bank

Table 1.6 GHI overall index in the MENA region

	GHS index: overall			GHS category: sufficient and robust health system		
	Regional rank	World rank	Score	Regional rank	World rank	Score
Qatar	1	49	48.7	3	60	42.4
Saudi Arabia	2	61	44.9	5	66	40.7
Jordan	3	66	42.8	1	52	47.1
UAE	4	80	39.6	12	123	19.5
Oman	5	81	39.6	8	91	28.6
Kuwait	6	88	36.8	2	59	42.5
Iran	7	90	36.5	6	70	39.4
Bahrain	8	92	36.3	4	63	41.2
Morocco	9	108	33.6	7	86	30.8
Lebanon	10	111	33.4	9	113	21.6
Tunisia	11	123	31.5	18	161	13
Sudan	12	152	28.3	19	164	12.8
Egypt	13	153	28	13	130	18.8
Algeria	14	163	26.2	14	151	15
Mauritania	15	163	26.2	10	117	21
Libya	16	172	25.3	17	161	13
Djibouti	17	173	25.2	15	155	14
Iraq	18	177	24	11	122	20.2
Syria	19	192	16.7	16	159	13.4
Yemen	20	193	16.1	20	167	12

Source: Global Health Security Index: Building Collective Action and Accountability, October 2019 (https://www.ghsindex.org/wp-content/uploads/2019/10/2019-Global-Health-Security-Index.pdf).

estimate, the number of new poor living below the middle-income poverty line of $5.50 per day will increase by 13 million in 2020 (Lakner et al., 2021). Lakner et al. (2020) estimated that 35 million people would fall into extreme poverty in the MENA region based on the growth forecast from April 2020 below the $1.90-a-day poverty line.

Additionally, prior to the COVID-19 crisis, the MENA region had one of the highest unemployment rates in the world, with over 4.68 million jobless in 2019 (ILO, 2020). Additionally, it is estimated that the pandemic will result in the loss of 1.7 million jobs by 2020 and a 1.2 percentage point increase in the unemployment rate (UNESCWA, 2020). According to the ILO's nowcasting model, working hours in the Arab region decreased by an estimated 2.2% in the first quarter of 2020 (equivalent to approximately 3 million full-time jobs assuming a 48-hour workweek) when compared to the pre-crisis period, namely the fourth quarter of 2019. For the second quarter of 2020, comparable estimates indicate a much sharper decline, with a loss of 19.5% of hours worked in comparison to the previous pre-crisis quarter; this equates to 23 million full-time jobs. For the third quarter of 2020, it is estimated that 12.8% of working hours will be lost, equating to 15 million full-time jobs (UNESCWA, 2021). Additionally, lockdown measures to contain the spread of the COVID-19 virus have had a significant impact on 89% of all informal workers in the region.

Pandemic Inequality

COVID-19 exposed and exacerbated inequality within and between MENA countries in a heinous manner. Throughout MENA, existing inequalities in the enjoyment of economic and social rights, as well as an entrenched culture of discrimination, resulted in certain groups of people being disproportionately affected by the pandemic, including people with disabilities, the elderly, refugees, migrant workers, and women. Numerous migrant workers and refugees are already at risk of contracting COVID-19 as a result of overcrowding in labor camps in Bahrain, Jordan, Kuwait, Lebanon, Oman, Qatar, Saudi Arabia, and the UAE (Amnesty, 2022).

Digital Divide

The pandemic is hastening technological change, shifting businesses and schools toward remote work and education, and increasing pressure on regional governments to ensure that their populations have regular and consistent Internet access at an affordable price (Xiao and Fan, 2020). However, lockdowns and social distancing measures have demonstrated how unequal Internet access in the MENA region has a detrimental effect on educational outcomes and economic opportunities for underprivileged groups such as women and rural populations. For instance, approximately 60% of students in Lebanon "either do not have a computer or must share one with at least three other family members" (World Bank, 2021b).

Even though 95% of people in the MENA region live within the range of at least a 3G mobile Internet signal, the International Telecommunications Union estimates that only 66% of people in the region used the Internet in 2021: an increase of 11% from 2019. Around 66% of people in general and 73% of young people in the MENA region were estimated to have used the Internet in 2020 (ITU, 2021). While only 42% of MENA rural households have access to the Internet, only 34% of rural residents do as well. According to the World Bank, school closures have already cost MENA students an average of 0.6 years of education (Kadi, 2021). As a result, the MENA region's digital divide will have a real-world impact on education and recovery.

Gender Inequality

Female healthcare and social service workers are exposed to greater risks of infection in the MENA region as compared to their male counterparts. Women will be forced to take on more unpaid care work as a result of government efforts to contain the spread of the pandemic, including homeschooling their children and caring for the sick and elderly (OECD, 2020). In addition, the pandemic may have a disproportionate impact on the dropout rates of girls (UNESCO, 2020). UN Women estimates that women in the MENA region will lose 700,000 jobs as a result of the epidemic (UN Women, 2020). In addition, more than 60% of women in the MENA region are informally employed in unregistered jobs that lack basic social or legal protection and employment benefits (ILO, 2018). Working longer hours and more days a week, women in Egypt's informal sector earn on average half the number of their male counterparts (AFDB, 2016). While the gender gap in mobile ownership increased from 8% to 9% between 2017 and 2020, the gender gap in mobile Internet use fluctuated during the same period, according to the GSM Association (but decreased slightly to 17%). Sixty-three million women in MENA do not have access to mobile Internet, which is the most common way for people to access online content (GSMA, 2021). Consequently, the pandemic's impact on women's employment, education, and financial security will be greater than that on men.

Freedom of Expression

As is often the case during times of war, freedom of expression is frequently the first casualty of the current crisis (Emerson, 1968). Governments throughout the world have enacted new policies aimed at combating misinformation or stepped-up enforcement of existing rules in the name of public health during the pandemic's course (Kaye, 2020). Governments throughout MENA have fully seized the opportunity to expand their powers, ostensibly to combat the burgeoning pandemic. They used the pandemic as an excuse to tighten their stranglehold on free expression, including prosecuting individuals who posted comments on social media criticizing government responses to the pandemic for spreading "false news" (Amnesty, 2021). Tunisia, for example, saw protests against worsening economic hardship met with disproportionate unlawful force and widespread arrests following months of lockdowns. The Egyptian government launched an arrest and intimidation campaign against medical professionals and others who spoke out against the regime's failing efforts to contain and conceal the virus's spread (Dunne, 2020). Algeria and Morocco's authorities declared a state of emergency and arrested or prosecuted those who voiced legitimate criticism about the pandemic. Moroccan authorities used a new health emergency law to prosecute human rights activists and citizen journalists for criticizing the government's handling of the pandemic. Over 25,000 Moroccans, many of them government critics, have been charged with violating the country's state of emergency, which was imposed on March 20 to aid in the fight against the coronavirus (Dunne, 2020). Jordan's government arrested 1,000 teachers as part of a crackdown on the Jordanian Teachers Syndicate, acting under the guise of emergency laws enacted to combat the coronavirus (Safi and Al-Tahat, 2020).

Omicron Wave

In mid-2022, when this book went to press, several countries in the MENA region are in partial lockdown, travel bans, lockdowns, and vaccine mandates to contain the Omicron strain of COVID-19, with many hoping that restrictions and vaccinations will begin to have an effect. Additional COVID-19 outbreaks, social unrest, high debt levels in some economies, and conflict in the MENA region could jeopardize economic activity and social stability. With less than two-fifths of MENA's population fully vaccinated, a significant risk exists (World Bank, 2022). Additionally, the rapid spread of Omicron may jeopardize regional food security by forcing migration, reducing labor productivity, and increasing the likelihood of conflict. Additionally, uncertainties and obstacles continue to loom over the region's potential economic recovery. Each country's situation is unique in that it varies according to its level of exposure to oil price fluctuations and its response to the pandemic via vaccine rollout. Significant asymmetries emerged during labor market recovery, and the region continues to face common challenges, including high unemployment, particularly among young people, and inadequate social protection. We are confronted with a critical issue: Is pandemic public policy effective? How will disparate approaches to public health affect the rate of economic and public health recovery and reopening? Has the pandemic of COVID-19 fundamentally altered public policy practices? How long can countries bear the hardships of curtailed education and punitive economic consequences associated with precautions taken to combat the coronavirus? What are the critical issues that policymakers should address to facilitate a rapid and sustained socioeconomic recovery? Will policymakers commit the necessary resources and reforms to avert future public health crises? What can the MENA region expect in the post-COVID era? Which major opportunities for growth and reform exist, and which major risks exist?

The pandemic is a game-changer for governments in the region, highlighting the need for robust governance strategies to address turbulent problems and highlighting the importance of public sector reforms to support robust governance of turbulence (Ansell et al., 2020). Post-COVID public management theory should incorporate our current perspective on public governance. Weible et al. (2020) identified ten perspectives on the COVID-19 pandemic's implications for policy sciences: policymaking; crisis response and management; global policymaking and transnational administration; policy networks; implementation and administration; scientific and technical expertise; emotions; narratives and messaging; learning; and policy success and failure. Additionally, Dunlop et al. (2020) examined seven analytical themes that merit increased attention in the post-pandemic era: policy design and instruments; policy learning; public service and its constituents; organizational capacity; public governance; administrative traditions; and public sector reforms in multi-level governance.

The post-pandemic era is likely to remain complex, with difficult questions that must be addressed before moving beyond the COVID-19 pandemic's previous phases. The stage has been set for this transition, but the months ahead will be occupied by decisions on the aforementioned issues, which will have a significant impact on how recovery looks and feels.

Overview of the Book

The chapters in this volume are structured around MENA governments' responses to the pandemic. Some of the chapters present new empirical findings; others provide critical reviews. Each chapter begins with a broad overview of the topic and goals of the chapter, presents background research on the topic from the international literature, provides new empirical data or reviews empirical studies suggests implications for policy and practice, and ends with implications for understanding the future of policy science. A brief description of each chapter follows.

First, Anis Ben Brik describes social protection and labor market responses to the COVID-19 pandemic in six Arab Gulf states: Saudi Arabia, Qatar, Bahrain, Kuwait, Oman, and the UAE. Based on a comprehensive set of social protection and labor market measures, using data from the global COVID-19 SPJ Policy Inventory, a total of 111 social protection measures have been implemented by Gulf states. Social assistance measures in the form of cash transfers, food, vouchers, and utility and financial obligation support followed by labor market policies in the form of wage subsidies, labor regulations, activation measures were the most prevalent responses used by the Gulf states. Labor regulatory flexibility targeting migrant workers was the most widely used labor market policy. The chapter shows an important aspect of the social protection responses to COVID-19 in the Gulf region is a shift from targeted interventions to providing universal support. However, the pandemic highlighted systemic gaps in social protection systems and has exposed and magnified some of the critical social protection challenges in the region. Expanding the social insurance system to provide more support to migrant workers could be an important pillar of social protection policies in Gulf countries. This is crucial for the Gulf region to weather its current challenges as well as future crises. In the longer span, effective structural transformation, legislative and policy reforms, including universal safety net and welfare innovation should be pursued.

Next, Diana Galeeva examines responses to COVID-19 in the UAE and Qatar. The chapter applies a neo-realist approach to International Relations theory to analyze small GCC states' responses. The chapter shows how the political status of the small GCC states has transformed globally, due to state characteristics and the actions implemented by their policymakers. The author argues that, in contrast to the neo-realist view, the GCC states, as demonstrated in the case studies of the UAE and Qatar, tackled the pandemic more effectively and have reported lower numbers of infections and consequently deaths. At the same time, wealth served as a vital power tool for offering foreign aid to both 'strong' and 'weak' states. In other words, such unprecedented events can provide an opportunity for policymakers to implement active foreign policies and even power projections. Overall, the pandemic, through the lens of foreign aid, has underlined the emergence of the UAE, particularly, and to a lesser extent, Qatar, on the global stage as potentially 'strong' states.

Nejla Ben Mimoune examines the institutional and policy journey against COVID-19 in Tunisia and Jordan. The chapter shows that the two countries' initial responses to COVID-19 were considered among the most effective in the region. Through national lockdowns, the two countries initially succeeded in containing the outbreak and flattening the first curve by early May 2020, with fatality rates that were comparable to global leaders such as Australia and New Zealand. However, such measures had serious economic repercussions in both countries, which pushed the two governments toward lifting all restrictions prematurely. The authors argue that Jordan and Tunisia continue to struggle to find the right balance between implementing measures to halt the pandemic and limiting its economic repercussions. Tunisia lacks a governance structure and e-governance, particularly in the health and education system. Several issues, regarding COVID-19 tracking and vaccine registration, had surfaced, while classes had been often disrupted with no online learning system in place since the start of the outbreak. The public healthcare system in Jordan lacks capacity and financial resources. The authors call for better governance and resources when dealing with refugees and asylum seekers, along with equal response among the different nationalities.

Lucia Ardovini addresses resilient authoritarianism and global pandemics in terms of the impact that the outbreak of COVID-19 has had on Egyptian society and institutions, focusing on how state responses to the pandemics shed light on ongoing attempts to further institutionalize authoritarianism in the country. The chapter shows that the Egyptian regime's attempts to shift the attention away from the reality of the pandemic by accusing its political opponents of misinformation and further cracking down on media and freedom of speech have wielded the opposite results and rather generated renewed attention to the inadequacy of state institution. The author argues that the discontent generated by the regime's inadequate response to COVID-19 had a direct impact on patterns of social transformation and unrest in the countries, which are likely to bear drastic implications for both policy and practice inside the country.

Ali Maleki and Najmoddin Yazdi focus on Iran's responses and challenges during the pandemic. The chapter examines a bottom-up citizen-driven response to the pandemic that focuses on decentralizing crisis management, enhancing public participation, mobilizing public resources, and the role of faith. Based on semi-structured interviews, the chapter shows that the proactive citizen-driven responses to the pandemic have historically been shaped by the people's collective memory and the centuries-old culture of help. The authors describe challenges of bottom-up responses such as the lack of information; ineffective coordination and cooperation; government dysfunctionality; lack of specialization and learning; and lack of empowerment and provision of root response to needs.

Alhafad Nouini and Abdelhakim Aboullouz's chapter explores how the state of emergency has affected rights and freedom of expression in Morocco and Tunisia. The chapter shows that both countries are still lacking in terms of constitutional protections for free expression, and fundamental rights and freedoms in general. The systems of governance in Morocco and Tunisia, especially their executive authorities and security apparatuses, still engage in authoritarian practices and do not shy away from exploiting any extraordinary or exceptional situation to further consolidate their power and reach. Government authorities in Morocco and Tunisia arrested journalists and citizens simply for expressing their views and also attempted to restrict this right by legislating draconian laws. The authors argue that the two countries used the pandemic as a pretext to consolidate the authoritarianism of their security apparatuses and to grant the executive ruling authority more powers against all other branches of governance.

Hamid Ait El Caid poses the question "why and under what conditions do policy-makers agree on what policies?". Using the method of most similar systems design, the chapter describes government responses, testing, social distancing measures, public health, and economic measures, and vaccination in three North African countries sharing similar cultural and socioeconomic characteristics. The chapter shows that while the three countries implemented similar responses to the pandemic, the difference between the three countries lies in the structural and social-relational aspects which produced different policy outcomes. The author argues that collaborative, multi-actors-based policy and consultation-based policy is critical to effective crisis management to curb infections and mitigate socioeconomic impacts.

Andreas Rechkemmer, Ozcan Ozturk, Anis Ben Brik, and Leslie A. Pal's chapter adds a dimension of tracking policy responses. The chapter describes government policies and measures in the fields of public health, economic and fiscal, and social policy across 12 MENA countries: Algeria, Egypt, Jordan, Lebanon, Morocco, Tunisia, and the six Gulf Cooperation Council (GCC) states (Bahrain, Kuwait, Oman, Qatar, Saudi Arabia, and the UAE). The chapter situates this policy tracker in the wider landscape of policy metrics and indexes, discusses its unique features, and presents key results on the policy responses to the pandemic in the MENA region – well beyond the actual field of sustainable development. The chapter shows that stringency, intensity, and sustainability of public health measures varied widely across the sample countries and over time; economic and fiscal policy measures looked essentially similar across the sample but varied greatly in terms of their intensity and the public investments made; and social policy measures, for the most part, appear to have been inadequate to the obvious social challenges linked to COVID-19 across the MENA region, with varying degrees.

Finally, the book concludes by providing a "future tense" for the MENA region, which will have to grapple with a new role for the state, changes in governance and social welfare. This final chapter argues the pandemic shock will remain with us, reverberating through theory and practice for years. That shock is not entirely the shock of the new. The pandemic did change the policy landscape in important ways, but it amplified trends and tendencies that pre-dated it or will sharpen and infect existing debates and disputes. A clear example is securitization – governments were already tracking and monitoring their citizens. The pandemic forced the creation of new tracking apps, more intense policing, and monitoring and lockdown control over entire societies.

Conclusion

The pandemic is both a rupture and an opportunity, amplifying fragility, uncertainty, and complexity while also pointing to potential solutions. The academic and scientific field of policy sciences had grown significantly in recent years, as evidenced by the global spread of policy programs, the explosion of journals and research, and the establishment of a stable core of accepted frameworks and conventional debates (Ben Brik and Pal, 2021). Governments' demand for policy advice and expertise had increased as well, and "capacity building" and "innovation" were at the forefront of every public sector reform agenda.

COVID-19 is the epitome of a disruptive agent. As the chapter summaries above demonstrate, it amplified existing wicked problems while also emphasizing the importance of global governance and evidence-based policy design. As we note in our concluding chapter, the pandemic has brought to light fundamental issues of governance and democracy, the balance of local and global interests, persistent inequalities, and a variety of pre-existing fragilities in the MENA region over the last decade.

By the time this book is published, it may very well be that the pandemic will be behind us. Vaccines will be administered across the region. MENA economies will revive, travel will resume, and people will seize the "normal". From a public policy perspective, however, COVID-19 was a near-death experience and street test for governments in the region.

Overall, the extent to which MENA countries recover in 2022 will depend on policy choices. As previously stated, vaccine access will be critical to recovery. Gulf countries that are less reliant on foreign debt and can afford to provide stronger fiscal stimulus, a high vaccination rate, and protection against future shocks will have a better chance of delivering a faster recovery than poorer nations. The imperative for cross-border collaboration is stronger than ever. Adopting a common desire for sustainable growth and prosperity will ensure the renaissance's success. Today's citizens in the

MENA region demand human rights alongside economic opportunity and democratization. It depends on whether MENA governments have the vision and political will to create a new world order that is not only equitable but also establishes the political, economic, and social conditions necessary to manage future pandemics at a potentially lower social and economic cost to all (Dorsey, 2020). The MENA region's renaissance will require new ways of doing things rather than relying on the same old habits that have brought the region to its knees. It will take political leadership with the foresight necessary to transform the region into one that is more inclusive and resilient – and the time to act is now.

References

AFDB. (2016). *Addressing informality in Egypt*. African Development Bank (AfDB), Abidjan, Ivory Coast. https://www.afdb.org/fileadmin/uploads/afdb/Documents/Publications/Working_paper_-_Addressing_informality_in_Egypt.pdf

Amnesty. (2021). *GCC: Flawed laws exploited in pandemic to further crush freedom of expression*. Amnesty International, London, UK. https://www.amnesty.org/en/latest/news/2020/10/gcc-flawed-laws-exploited-in-pandemic-to-further-crush-freedom-of-expression/

Amnesty. (2022). *MENA: COVID-19 amplified inequalities and was used to further ramp up repression*. Amnesty International, London, UK. https://www.amnesty.org/en/latest/news/2021/04/mena-covid-19-amplified-inequalities-and-was-used-to-further-ramp-up-repression/

Ansell, C., Sørensen, E., & Torfing, J. (2020). The COVID-19 pandemic as a game-changer for public administration and leadership? The need for robust governance responses to turbulent problems. *Public Management Review*, 23(7), 949–960. https://doi.org/10.1080/14719037.2020.1820272

Balkhi, B., Alshayban, D., & Alotaibi, N. M. (2021). Impact of healthcare expenditures on healthcare outcomes in the Middle East and North Africa (MENA) region: A cross-country comparison, 1995–2015. *Frontiers in Public Health*, 8. https://doi.org/10.3389/fpubh.2020.624962

Ben Brik, A., & A. Pal, L. (2021). Introduction: Futures, now and then. In *The Future of the Policy Sciences*, Edward Elgar Publishing, pp. 1–8. https://doi.org/10.4337/9781800376489.00008

Dorsey, J. (2020). Turning Gulf security upside down. *Middle East Insights, 238*. https://mei.nus.edu.sg/wp-content/uploads/2020/07/Insight-238-James-Dorsey-1.pdf

Dunlop, C. A., Ongaro, E., & Baker, K. (2020). Researching COVID-19: A research agenda for public policy and administration scholars. *Public Policy and Administration, 35*(4), 365–383. https://doi.org/10.1177/0952076720939631

Dunne, C. W. (2020). *North African autocrats use the pandemic to expand power, settle scores*. Arab Center, Washington, DC. https://arabcenterdc.org/resource/north-african-autocrats-use-the-pandemic-to-expand-power-settle-scores/

Emerson, T. I. (1968). Freedom of expression in wartime. *University of Pennsylvania Law Review, 116*(6), 975. https://doi.org/10.2307/3311117

ESCWA. (2021). *Towards a productive and inclusive path: Job creation in the Arab Region*. United Nations Economic and Social Commission for Western Asia.

https://publications.unescwa.org/projects/jcar/sdgs/pdf/en/21-00024_Job%20
Creation%20in%20the%20Arab%20Region_IDigital.pdf

Gatti, R. V., Lederma D., Fan, R. Y., Hatefi A., Nguyen H., Sautman A., Sax, J. M., & Wood, C. A. (2021). *MENA public healthcare systems: Building resilience for future emergencies*. https://theforum.erf.org.eg/2021/11/11/mena-public-healthcare-systems-building-resilience-future-emergencies/

GHSI. (2019). *Global health security index: Building collective action and accountability*. GHS Index. https://www.ghsindex.org/wp-content/uploads/2019/10/2019-Global-Health-Security-Index.pdf

GSMA. (2021). *Connected women: The mobile gender gap report 2021*. Global System for Mobile Communications Association. https://www.gsma.com/r/wp-content/uploads/2021/07/The-Mobile-Gender-Gap-Report-2021.pdf

Hoogeveen, J. G., & Lopez-Acevedo G. (2021). *Distributional impacts of COVID-19 in the Middle East and North Africa region*. *MENA development report*. World Bank, Washington, DC. https://openknowledge.worldbank.org/bitstream/handle/10986/36618/9781464817762.pdf

ILO. (2018). *Women and Men in the informal economy: A statistical picture*. International Labour Office, Geneva. https://www.ilo.org/wcmsp5/groups/public/—dgreports/—dcomm/documents/publication/wcms_626831.pdf

ILO. (2020). *COVID-19: Labour market impact and policy response in the Arab States*. International Labour Organization, Beirut. https://www.ilo.org/wcmsp5/groups/public/—arabstates/—ro-beirut/documents/briefingnote/wcms_744832.pdf

ITU. (2021). *Measuring digital development: Facts and figures, 2021*. International Telecommunication Union, Geneva. https://www.itu.int/en/ITU-D/Statistics/Documents/facts/FactsFigures2021.pdf

Kadi, S. (2021). *Post-covid-19, Arab countries need new approaches to education, U.N. Official says*. Al-Fanar Media. https://www.al-fanarmedia.org/2021/05/post-covid-19-arab-countries-need-new-approaches-to-education-u-n-official-says/

Kaye, D. (2020). *Disease pandemics and the freedom of opinion and expression*. Report of the U.N. Hum. Its. Council on its Forty-Fourth Session, June 15–July 3, 2020, 48–49, U.N. Doc. A/HRC/44/49 (2020). United Nations: Geneva, Switzerland.

Lakner, C., Mahler, D. G., Negre M., & Prydz, E. B. (2020). *How much does reducing inequality matter for global poverty?* World Bank, Poverty and Equity Global Practice Group. https://documents1.worldbank.org/curated/en/765601591733806023/pdf/How-Much-Does-Reducing-Inequality-Matter-for-Global-Poverty.pdf

Lakner, C., Yonzan, N., Mahler, D. G., Aguilar, A. C., & Wu, H. (2021). *Updated estimates of the impact of COVID-19 on global poverty: Looking back at 2020 and the outlook for 2021*. World Bank Blogs. https://blogs.worldbank.org/opendata/updated-estimates-impact-covid-19-global-poverty-looking-back-2020-and-outlook-2021

OECD. (2020). *COVID-19 crisis in the MENA region: Impact on gender equality and policy responses*. https://www.oecd.org/coronavirus/policy-responses/covid-19-crisis-in-the-mena-region-impact-on-gender-equality-and-policy-responses-ee4cd4f4/

Safi, M., & Al-Tahat, J. (2020). *Jordan arrests 1,000 teachers in crackdown on the union*. The Guardian. https://www.theguardian.com/world/2020/aug/19/jordan-arrests-1000-teachers-in-crackdown-on-union

UNDP. (2020). *Compounding crises: Will COVID-19 and lower oil prices lead to a new development paradigm in the Arab Region?* United Nations Development

Programme, New York. https://www.arabdevelopmentportal.com/sites/default/files/publication/compounding_crisis_undp_feb07-2021_combined_v3_2.pdf

UNDP, & OPHI. (2021). *Global Multidimensional Poverty Index 2021 Unmasking disparities by ethnicity, ca2ste, and gender.* United Nations Development Programme and Oxford Poverty and Human Development Initiative. https://hdr.undp.org/sites/default/files/2021_mpi_report_en.pdf

UNESCO. (2020). *Covid-19 school closures around the world will hit girls hardest.* https://en.unesco.org/news/covid-19-school-closures-around-world-will-hit-girls-hardest.

UNESCWA. (2020). *COVID-19 economic cost to the Arab Region.* United Nations Economic and Social Commission for Western Asia. https://archive.unescwa.org/sites/www.unescwa.org/files/escwa-covid-19-economic-cost-arab-region-en.pdf

UN Women. (2020). *The impact of COVID-19 on gender equality in the Arab States.* https://www2.unwomen.org/-/media/field%20office%20arab%20states/attachments/publications/2020/04/impact%20of%20covid%20on%20gender%20equality%20-%20policy%20brief.pdf?la=en&vs=4414

Weible, C. M., Nohrstedt, D., Cairney, P., Carter, D. P., Crow, D. A., Durnová, A. P., Heikkila, T., Ingold, K., McConnell, A., & Stone, D. (2020). COVID-19 and the policy sciences: Initial reactions and perspectives. *Policy Sciences, 53*(2), 225–241. https://doi.org/10.1007/s11077-020-09381-4

WHO. (2021a). *Nursing and midwifery personnel, Global Health Observatory data repository.* https://apps.who.int/gho/data/node.main.HWFGRP_0040?lang=en

WHO. (2021b). *World Health Organization (WHO), Medical Doctors, Global Health Observatory data repository.* https://apps.who.int/gho/data/node.main.HWFGRP_0020?lang=en

World Bank. (2021a). *Lebanon sinking (to the top 3). Lebanon Economic Monitor.* https://openknowledge.worldbank.org/bitstream/handle/10986/35626/Lebanon-Economic-Monitor-Lebanon-Sinking-to-the-Top-3.pdf?sequence=1&isAllowed=y

World Bank. (2021b). *Life expectancy at birth, total (years) – the Middle East & North Africa.* World Bank Open Data | Data. https://data.worldbank.org/indicator/SP.DYN.LE00.IN?locations=ZQ

World Bank. (2022). *Global economic prospects: The Middle East and North Africa, January 2022.* https://thedocs.worldbank.org/en/doc/cb15f6d7442eadedf75bb-95c4fdec1b3-0350012022/related/Global-Economic-Prospects-January-2022-Regional-Overview-MENA.pdf

Worldometer. (2022). *COVID-19 coronavirus pandemic.* https://www.worldometers.info/coronavirus.

Xiao Y., & Fan Z. (2020). *10 tech trends getting us through the COVID-19 pandemic.* World Economic Forum. https://www.weforum.org/agenda/2020/04/10-technology-trends-coronavirus-covid19-pandemic-robotics-telehealth/ads/2019/10/2019-Global-Health- Security-Index.pdf).

2 Social Protection Responses in the Arabian Gulf Region

Anis Ben Brik

Introduction

The COVID-19 pandemic has posed unprecedented health and economic security challenges for the Gulf states – Saudi Arabia, Oman, Kuwait, Bahrain, Qatar, and the UAE – necessitating swift and comprehensive responses. The UAE reported the first COVID-19 case on January 29, 2020, followed by Bahrain, Oman, and Kuwait (February 24), Qatar (February 29), and Saudi Arabia (March 2, 2020). As of November 30, 2020, the COVID-19 pandemic had confirmed nearly 1 million cases and nearly 20,000 deaths (Worldmeters.info, 2020). Gulf states have taken unprecedented precautionary measures, including indefinite curfews and the isolation of major cities, to mitigate the pandemic's effects. On March 18 and March 20, 2020, Oman and Bahrain implemented lockdowns and border closures, respectively. The Kingdom of Saudi Arabia (KSA) suspended transportation services on March 21, implemented a night curfew on March 23, and a 24-hour curfew in early April 2020. Kuwait implemented a 24-hour curfew on March 22, 2020 and ordered the immediate closure of all schools and colleges. By March 25, 2020, Qatar implemented a complete lockdown and work/study from home order. The UAE suspends public transportation on March 26 but does not implement a complete curfew until April 4, 2020. These government actions have impacted all segments of the population, including the poor, the elderly, disabled individuals, students, children, migrant workers, and women (Alamri et al., 2020; Alenazi et al., 2020; Algahtani et al., 2021; Alkhamees et al., 2020; Alshehri et al., 2020; Alyami et al., 2020; Alyoubi et al., 2021; Balkhi et al., 2020; El Keshky et al., 2021; Iqbal and Tayyab, 2020; Sonbol et al., 2021).

Social protection was critical in responding to the 2008 financial, food, and energy crises (Grosh et al., 2013), and it has been elevated as a COVID-19 response tool. Social protection systems (social insurance, social assistance, and labor market policies) are critical in the context of the COVID-19 pandemic because they are designed to address the crisis's temporary spikes in poverty and unemployment by providing social assistance to the poor and social insurance to working people during times of unemployment (e.g.,

DOI: 10.4324/9781003266259-2

sickness, maternity leave, or retirement) (Devereux, 2021). Additionally, social protection measures may be used to eliminate financial barriers to essential testing and health care; to enable infected workers to comply with confinement measures without incurring income losses; to assist households, particularly those in informal sectors, in meeting basic needs during periods of reduced economic activity and growing unemployment, thereby ensuring food security and averting a significant decline in living standards; and to assist businesses in retaining employees (ILO, 2020a).

In comparison to previous global crises, the unprecedented social protection responses since the onset of COVID-19 includes shock-responsive programs and platforms for horizontal expansion (registering more beneficiaries) or vertical expansion (temporarily increasing benefits) – which have recently gained traction in several countries (Gentilini et al., 2020). Additionally, the social protection adjustments and innovative practices implemented since the crisis's inception raise questions and provide insight into the effectiveness of crisis response. While the majority of social protection responses in many countries are intended to be temporary, they also have long-term policy and system implications (Gentilini et al., 2020). Notably, such crisis responses have been accompanied by broader calls to "build better in the direction of a 'new normal,' with the establishment of a new social contract at the center of the recovery effort" (Bastagli and Lowe, 2021). As such, the COVID-19 crisis served as a wake-up call to strengthen social protection and is providing renewed impetus to address policy gaps and limitations throughout the crisis and beyond, to assist countries in becoming more prepared for future crises. This article examines the social protection and labor market responses to COVID-19 in six Gulf states against this backdrop.

Methodology

This chapter draws on data collected by the global COVID-19 SPJ Policy Inventory, MENA tracker database, and ILO database for social protection responses. The COVID-19 Social Protection and Jobs (SPJ) Policy Inventory builds on and expands on data collected by Gentilini et al. (2020), who detailed social protection policies implemented by countries worldwide since the pandemic's start. It strengthens the labor market component by including demand-side labor market policies and by providing additional detail on social protection and labor market programs relevant to the COVID-19 context. Gentilini et al. (2020) collected qualitative and quantitative data on each policy, including the benefit's name, description, start and end dates, targeting mechanism, intended and actual beneficiaries, and, where available, expenditures. SPJ policies are included in the COVID-19 SPJ policy inventory on both the supply side and demand side of the labor market. On the supply side of the labor market, it encompasses policies that assist workers in maintaining their income and employment, such as public works, income tax reduction, training and placement assistance, and unemployment benefits. On the demand side of the labor market, it encompasses policies that assist businesses in surviving and retaining employees, such as firm liquidity or entrepreneurship support. Additionally, the inventory reflects changes in regulations governing the employer-employee relationship during the pandemic. While these labor regulations affect both workers and businesses, they are implemented by businesses and are thus considered demand-side interventions for this analysis. The data collection period was March 2020 to October 31, 2021. The mapping supplemented Gentilini et al.'s already exhaustive collection of social protection and job programs with policies related to labor demand (2020). Additionally, the paper is based on a comprehensive review of the literature and a report on shock-responsive SP in the Gulf region. Additional data on social protection responses were gathered from the websites of government entities, peer-reviewed articles, and grey literature in English and Arabic.

Social Protection and Labor Market Responses in the Gulf Countries

Gulf states have scaled up social protection in response to COVID-19. A total of 111 social protection measures were adopted in the six Gulf states between March 2020 and October 2021. Saudi Arabia has the largest share of SP programs (29% of all measures), followed by the UAE (23%), Kuwait (14%), Bahrain (13%), Oman (12%), and Qatar (10%) (see Table 2.1).

Across the 111 measures mapped, social assistance (47%) in the form of cash transfers, food, vouchers, and utility waivers & financial obligation support was the most frequent SP component used in the response by Gulf states, followed by labor market policies in the form of wage subsidies, labor regulations, and activation measures (33%). Social insurance measures in the form of paid sick leave, healthcare insurance, unemployment insurance scheme, and social security contributions were the least frequent measures (19%). Table 2.2 shows in greater detail the social protection categories adopted by Gulf states. In this regard, it is noticeable that UAE has the

Table 2.1 Social protection responses to COVID-19, by country (number, % of all measures), March 2020–October 2021

Countries	Number of responses		Percentage
Saudi Arabia		32	29
Qatar	11	10	
Oman	13	12	
Bahrain	14	13	
Kuwait	15	14	
UAE	26	23	

Table 2.2 Social protection responses to COVID-19 by category, by country (number, % of all measures), March 2020–October 2021

Countries	Social assistance	Social insurance	Labor market
Saudi Arabia	11 (10%)	6 (5%)	15 (14%)
Qatar	4 (4%)	2 (2%)	5 (5%)
Oman	6 (5%)	3 (3%)	4 (4%)
Bahrain	7 (6%)	2 (2%)	5 (5%)
Kuwait	8 (7%)	3 (3%)	4 (4%)
UAE	16 (14%)	5 (5%)	5 (5%)

Table 2.3 Social protection responses to COVID-19 by instrument, by country (number, % of all measures), March 2020–October 2021

	Number of instruments	Percentage
Cash transfers	10	9
In-kind transfers	15	14
Utility waivers & financial obligation support	27	24
Paid sick leave	7	6
Health insurance	7	6
Unemployment benefits	4	4
Social security contributions	3	3
Activation measures	4	4
Wage subsidies	11	10
Labor regulations and shorter work time arrangements	23	21

largest proportion of social assistance measures (14%) followed by Saudi Arabia (10%). The two countries also had the largest proportion of social insurance measures (5%, respectively). In addition, Saudi Arabia leads in labor market policies (14%) which can be explained by the high proportion of migrant workers in the labor market. Qatar has the smallest proportion of social assistance and social insurance (4% and 2%, respectively). Kuwait and Oman are lagging behind other Gulf countries in labor market measures (4%, respectively). Furthermore, while labor market measures were the most prevalent measure adopted by Saudi Arabia and Qatar (15 and 5 measures, respectively), social assistance was the most commonly used measure in the UAE, Kuwait, Bahrain, and Oman.

The most commonly used social protection instruments across Gulf states were utility waivers & financial obligation support (24%) followed by labor regulations and shorter work time arrangements (21%), as shown in Table 2.3. In-kind transfers and wage subsidies were also very widely used social protection instruments, in the Gulf region (14% and 10%, respectively). Cash transfers account for 9% of all measures in Gulf states. Furthermore, very few instruments such as paid sick leave, health insurance, unemployment benefits, and social security contributions were mapped in the Gulf region.

Options for Scaling up in Social Protection Measures

The implementation of social assistance measures included horizontal expansion – extending coverage to people previously uncovered either through existing programs or the creation of new interventions; implementation changes – the anticipation of payments/withdrawals, changes in the delivery modality, waivers of conditionality, and flexibilization of payment duties; vertical expansion – provides existing beneficiaries of SP programs with additional benefits, either by increasing the value of the assistance received through the program or by introducing new components to it; piggybacking – using elements of existing social protection programs while delivering a separate response; and refocusing – adjusting the social protection system to refocus assistance on groups most vulnerable to the shock (Bastagli, 2014).

As shown in Table 2.4, the most prevalent scale-up option was implementation changes (44%), followed by horizontal expansion by enrolling additional beneficiaries – the poor, people with disabilities, families, and elder people (23%). The vertical and horizontal expansion was also a popular scale-up option (11%). Only a few social protection programs were being scaled up based on the vertical expansion (7%). Only 4% of all measures were piggybacked on existing programs and five programs were refocusing – adjusting the social protection system to refocus assistance on groups most vulnerable to the shock (see Table 2.5). Moreover, except with Kuwait, most social protection measures were expanded through implementation changes in Saudi Arabia (11 measures), Qatar (five measures), Oman (seven measures), Bahrain (six measures), and UAE (ten measures). In Kuwait, most of the measures were expanded horizontally (seven measures).

Table 2.4 Implementation features of social assistance measures in response to COVID-19, by countries, March 2020–October 2021

	Saudi Arabia	Qatar	Oman	Bahrain	Kuwait	UAE	Total measure (%)
Vertical expansion only	3 (3%)	0	1 (1%)	2 (2%)	0	2 (2%)	8 (7%)
Implementation changes only	11 (10%)	5 (4%)	7 (6%)	6 (5%)	5 (4%)	10 (9%)	44 (44%)
Horizontal expansion only	8 (7%)	3 (3%)	2 (2%)	1 (1%)	7 (6%)	2 (2%)	23 (21%)
Vertical and horizontal expansion	2 (2%)	0	0	2 (2%)	3 (3%)	4 (4%)	11 (10%)
Vertical and implementation changes	0	2 (2%)	0	2 (2%)	0	2 (2%)	6 (5%)
Horizontal and implementation changes	4 (4%)	1 (1%)	0	0	0	1 (1%)	6 (5%)
Vertical, horizontal, and implementation changes	2 (2%)	0	0	0	0	2 (2%)	4 (4%)
Piggybacking	1 (1%)	1 (1%)	1 (1%)	0	0	1 (1%)	4 (4%)
Refocusing	1 (1%)	0	2 (2%)	1 (1%)	0	1 (1%)	5 (5%)

Coverage

Social protection measures have almost exclusively been implemented to support nationals (39%) including formal employees (23%), vulnerable individuals such as the poor, those with disabilities, prisoners' families, elderly people, pregnant women, widows, divorced women, orphans, those with chronic diseases, and breastfeeding women), and 7% of measures targeted poor and vulnerable households, as shown in Table 2.5. Although Gulf countries are in the process of phasing out universal social protection measures (28%), nearly half of the measured targeted exclusively citizens (47%) and a quarter of SP measures targeted migrant workers.

Social assistance was mostly universal measures targeting all affected individuals (23%), followed by measures targeting nationals (20%). Nevertheless, Gulf countries have not ruled out cash transfers to migrant workers, who are most affected by pandemic measures. Cash transfer programs adopted as social assistance were directed to exclusively citizens (9%), as shown in Table 2.6. In addition, utility waivers & financial obligation support have been expanded to target both citizens and migrant workers (12% and 6%, respectively). Moreover, in-kind transfers have targeted all affected individuals (9%).

Labor market policies have been geared towards benefiting migrant workers (16%) and nationals (15%). Most labor regulations and shorter work time arrangements adopted were directed to migrant workers (15%). In addition, most wage subsidies were targeting nationals (8%). Furthermore, social insurance measures have mostly targeted all affected individuals (10%). However, migrant workers were excluded from unemployment benefits, which has been having been geared towards benefiting nationals (4% of all measures).

Table 2.5 Target groups of social protection measures, by country (number, % of all measures), March 2020–October 2021

		Saudi Arabia	Qatar	Oman	Bahrain	Kuwait	UAE	Total measure (%)
Nationals	Formal employees	13 (12%)	1 (1%)	5 (4%)	2 (2%)	2 (2%)	2 (2%)	25 (23%)
	Poor and vulnerable households	2 (2%)	0	1 (1%)	2 (2%)	3 (3%)	0	8 (7%)
	Vulnerable individuals	3 (3%)	1 (1%)	0	0	4 (4%)	3 (3%)	11 (9%)
Migrant workers		6 (5%)	6 (5%)	3 (3%)	3 (3%)	3 (3%)	7 (6%)	28 (25%)
Universal		8 (7%)	4 (4%)	4 (4%)	7 (6%)	4 (4%)	12 (11%)	39 (35%)

Table 2.6 Target groups of social protection measures, by instruments (number, % of all measures), March 2020–October 2021

Category	Instruments	Coverage		
		Nationals	Migrant workers	Universal
Social assistance	Cash transfers	10 (9%)	0	
	In-kind transfers	4 (4%)	1 (1%)	10 (9%)
	Utility waivers & financial obligation support	13 (12%)	7 (6%)	6 (5%)
Social insurance	Paid sick leave	0	2 (2%)	5 (4%)
	Health insurance[a]	0	0	7 (6%)
	Unemployment benefits	4 (4%)	0	0
	Social security contributions	3 (3%)	0	0
Labor market	Activation measures	3 (3%)	1 (1%)	0
	Wage subsidies	9 (8%)	0	2 (2%)
	Labor regulations and shorter work time arrangements	5 (4%)	17 (15%)	2 (2%)

[a]Nationals have free healthcare.

Social Protection and Labor Market Measures

In the following subsections, each of the three social protection and labor market categories, social assistance, social insurance, and the labor market will be analyzed separately, with a focus on how the measures allowed temporary vertical or horizontal expansion of SP systems, and the adaptation of SP systems to the pandemic context.

Social Assistance Measures

The most commonly used social assistance instruments across the Gulf countries were utility waivers & financial obligation support in the form of waiving and postponing of tax payments: including residence visa renewal, exit, and return fees, dependents levies; and fees for hiring expatriates and obtaining visas for their dependents; and suspending rent payments (24% of all measures). Except for Kuwait, utility waivers & financial obligation support were the premier instrument adopted by Saudi Arabia, Oman, Bahrain, Qatar, and the UAE. In addition, in-kind transfers were also a very widely used social assistance instrument (14% of all measures), especially in Kuwait and UAE. Furthermore, cash transfers were the least adopted instrument in the Gulf region. Bahrain, Kuwait, and Saudi Arabia have the largest share of cash transfer programs (3% of all measures) (see Table 2.7).

The most common social assurance measures adopted by Gulf countries are discussed below.

Table 2.7 Social assistance measures, by instrument, by country (number, % of all measures), March 2020–October 2021

	Saudi Arabia	Qatar	Oman	Bahrain	Kuwait	UAE	Total
Cash transfers	3 (3%)	1 (1%)	0	3 (3%)	3 (3%)	0	10 (9%)
In-kind transfers	3 (3%)	0	2 (2%)	0	5 (5%)	5 (5%)	15 (14%)
Utility waivers & financial obligation support	5 (5%)	3 (3%)	4 (4%)	4 (4%)	0	11 (10%)	27 (24%)

Horizontal Shock-Response: Cash Transfer for Families

Cash transfers in Saudi Arabia came in the form of a new temporary one-off emergency cash transfer scheme to support beneficiaries and beneficiaries of social security in the amount of $267 for the family and $134 for the dependent. The Bahraini government provided direct aid to 17,000 families in need and doubled the monthly assistance for those registered in Social Affairs and the Royal Foundation for Humanitarian Action. Funds of $14.63 million for additional social security benefits were established. The Kuwaiti government provided on-off temporary cash transfers to widows, divorced women, orphans, and the elderly. In addition, low-income families received top-up financial assistance.

Community Fund

The Saudi and Kuwaiti governments appealed to a sense of national crisis and the need for collective action, partly as a way of depoliticizing the pandemic, has established a "community fund" which aims to mobilize societal efforts, direct them towards societal needs and priorities at this critical stage and to finance a set of community-based initiatives and projects to support the segments of society most in need and those most affected by this pandemic, including poor people, people with disabilities, widows, divorced women, prisoners' families, elderly people, workers in the minor professions, affected workers, needy students, those in need who are coming to the Kingdom for Umrah or to visit, and others. In Saudi Arabia, the community fund covers various fields, including relief, social, educational, health awareness, technical, service, housing, mosques, the Two Holy Places, and others. The fund was co-financed, with government contribution, donations solicited from the non-profit and private sectors, and individuals in addition. In Kuwait, the Fazaa El-Kuwait program, a public-private initiative in collaboration with NGOs/charities/volunteers, provided cash and in-kind transfers. As of May 30, 2020, $17.29 million was distributed via cash assistance to impacted families through rent payments, general cash assistance, and distribution of shopping carts.

In-Kind Transfers

Measures in this area include providing food baskets, cooked meals, and other necessities to vulnerable and underprivileged persons. Many initiatives in this area were private-public initiatives and timed during Ramadan.

The Saudi government used existing programs such as Ramadan Meals for horizontal expansion, as a way of scaling up support rapidly during a crisis. The 'Ramadan Iftar' initiative (Ramadan meals) is a national initiative funded by the social fund of the Ministry of Human Resources and Social Development and directed at those affected by the pandemic during the holy month of Ramadan. Benefits consist of hot or dry meals or food baskets, according to each category of beneficiaries, and the conditions of the curfew in each region. The government has also established a new emergency program (e.g., "Our Food One"), to distribute food baskets to the most vulnerable groups affected by the Coronavirus virus, from the poor, people with disabilities, widows, divorced women, prisoners' families, and the elderly). More than 142,000 food baskets were distributed to families in need, both citizens and residents alike.

The Omani government launched the "Salat Al Khair" initiative whereby food baskets composed of 19 essential food items were sold at a subsidized fixed cost of $23. Additionally, food baskets were delivered to vulnerable families during Ramadan 2020, via public donations which included in-kind donations from shopping centers. Lastly as of April 2020, 2,000 food baskets containing rice, wheat, oil, sugar, and other essential items were distributed to Omani and ex-pat families.

Kuwait's 'Fazaa El-Kuwait' program distributed shopping cards providing 331,273 food baskets, 495,123 meals, and 405,682 hand sanitizers. The Ministry of Social Affairs had provided in-kind assistance in the form of 307,605 food baskets benefiting 276,741 families and affected workers in quarantine; 393,858 sanitizers; 254,576 warm meals for hospitals, government entities, and quarantine locations. The Kuwaiti Red Crescent Society in partnership with the Ministry of Interior and Governorate distributed 1,500 food parcels and 1,500 milk cartons to workers and residents in Al-Jahra Governorate. Additionally, three months' worth of support/meals were provided for people living in nursing homes, workers of nursing homes, and those who need social care. General Authority for Disability Affairs – The 'Friends of PwD' team distributed 1,200 food baskets to persons with full disabilities.

UAE

The UAE government provided three months of food and essentials for 44,500 families. On April 19, 2020, the UAE launched a campaign, the '10 million meals', to support low-income families and individuals financially affected by the effects of the lockdowns and pandemics. The government in partnership with the private sector provided cooked meals from local restaurants to vulnerable families during Ramadan. Moreover, the "Meer" initiative was launched to provide senior citizens with food and essential services.

Housing

The Bahraini government provided temporary housing to migrant workers to reduce overcrowding and ease congestion.

The Kuwaiti government built temporary homes for nearly 25,000 migrant workers and provided basic income for the laborers to meet living costs.

Utility Waivers & Financial Obligation Support

Except for Kuwait, all the Gulf states provided waving of utility payments, delay in loan installment payments, and reduction in visa/residence fees.

Saudi Arabia

Saudi government waived payments temporarily for government-provided utilities – mainly electricity and rent – either for all citizens or foreign workers, for six months. Electricity consumers received a 30% discount for April and May 2020 bills. The government waived also loan installments due on all financing facilities extended to Saudi employees, without additional fees for three months. Another innovative intervention was a temporary suspension of fees for hiring expatriates and obtaining visas for their dependents including residence visa renewal fees, exit, and return visas. In addition, the government decided on the automatic extension of visas and residency permits (Iqamas) inside and outside of the country from March to September 2020, while traveling from/to Saudi Arabia was suspended. The Qatari government waived rental and utility fees for households and businesses until February 2022.

The Omani government accepted utility bill payments in information and extreme cases permitted delayed payments. The government provided the national fuel support card to low-wage Omani (expatriates excluded) workers in the private sector. Financial institutions were asked to postpone and reschedule the repayment of loans for employees that had their salaries reduced due to the pandemic. In addition, the government introduced measures in regard to tax payments: The 1% fee levied against taxes paid in installments was waived, and an additional 1% reduction in taxes due, was provided to all taxpayers that filed taxes for 2021 by the due date.

In Bahrain, the government forgave electricity and water payments for households and allocated $66.5 million towards exempting households from paying municipality fees for three months. Banks were requested to offer a six-month deferral of re-payments without interest or penalty and refrain from blocking customer accounts if they have lost their employment. Moreover, the Labor Market Regulatory Authority (LMRA) terminated monthly work fees and fees for issuing and renewing work permits, providing aggregated exemptions worth $149 million between April and June 2020.

The Kuwaiti government amended tenancy laws to stop evictions due to late payment. Persons living in the Zakat house were exempted from paying rent.

In the UAE, the government reduced water fees and subsidized electricity by 10% for three months. The Emirates Red Crescent Authority announced a new initiative called 'Among your Family' to reduce rent payments for existing tenants. In addition, the government passed a law requiring current employers to continue providing housing and general allowances for workers who have lost their jobs due to the pandemic until they leave the country or find another job. Moreover, the government postponed the payment of public housing loans for citizens working in the private sector for up to three months and halted penalty measures against late payments.

Social Insurance Measures

The most widely adopted social insurance measures were paid sick leave and healthcare insurance (14% of all measures). Only a few countries provided unemployment benefits (4% of all measures) and social security contributions (allowing firms to postpone the payment of their part of social security contributions as an easy way for governments to help businesses without having to make additional transactions or reallocating resources (3%). Qatar, Bahrain, and Kuwait have not ruled out unemployment benefits and Oman has not adopted paid sick leave measures. In addition, Saudi Arabia, Qatar, and Bahrain were lagging behind other countries in providing social security contributions. Kuwait has not provided health insurance (see Table 2.8).

The most common social insurance measures adopted by Gulf countries include:

Table 2.8 Social insurance measures, by instrument, by country (number, % of all measures), March 2020–October 2021

	Saudi Arabia	Qatar	Oman	Bahrain	Kuwait	UAE	Total
Paid sick leave	2 (2%)	1 (1%)		1 (1%)	1 (1%)	2 (2%)	7 (7%)
Health insurance	2 (2%)	1 (1%)	1 (1%)	1 (1%)		2 (2%)	7 (7%)
Unemployment benefits	2 (2%)		1 (1%)		1 (1%)		4 (4%)
Social security contributions			1 (1%)		1 (1%)	1 (1%)	3 (3%)

Paid Sick Leave

The Saudi government has provided two weeks of paid sick leave (additional to all usual leave entitlements under the labor law) to those with autoimmune disease, cancer, respiratory illness, chronic illnesses, and pregnant women or breastfeeding women as well as employees aged 55 years and above. In addition, the government allowed paid sick leave for private-sector workers in the private sector, including in case of self-quarantine.

The Kuwaiti government prohibited employees placed under quarantine from working and stressed that salaries for Kuwaiti and non-Kuwaiti staff will continue to be paid during any period of quarantine. Their absence from work will not impact their employment status. The duration is equivalent to the quarantine period.

In the UAE, the government has amended the law of Human Resources a regulation that any employee that is hospitalized or being in a quarantine period will be paid fully sick leave benefit. Also, a regulation has been set that a spouse of a sick employee will be paid fully during the period of an employee being hospitalized or allocated to a quarantine facility due to COVID-19. Moreover, the government has called on private-sector establishments to consider workers infected with COVID-19 as sick cases entitled to sick leave.

Health Insurance

In Saudi Arabia, the government offered free healthcare to all Saudi citizens and foreign workers, including workers in an irregular situation. In addition, the government mandated an automatic renewal of health insurance cards for six months, hence allowing families to make hospital and clinic visits.

In Qatar, the treatment for COVID-19 is provided to anyone free of charge – the possession of a health card and/or the Qatar ID is not necessary to be tested and/or receive treatment.

The Omani government expanded the services covered by the health insurance scheme, including medical tests and treatment costs for insured members with COVID-19 (both nationals and expatriates) under their medical insurance coverage. Additionally, for those without health insurance or sponsors, the government offered free treatment (for residents and citizens).

In Bahrain, the government covered the treatment expenses of COVID-19 patients, including testing and quarantine services, for all citizens and residents.

The UAE government provided full health coverage for all (Citizen, Resident, & Tourist) infected or who were exposed to COVID-19, during their treatment and quarantine period.

Unemployment Benefits

The Saudi government has provided unemployment insurance in the form of a three-month extension of support to Saudis working in the private sector affected by the pandemic. Moreover, the government provided monthly income support to jobseekers for 15 months. The unemployment benefits ranged from $534 to $200. In addition, the scheme provided beneficiaries with integrated support through training.

In Oman, workers contributing to the Public Authority for Social Insurance (PASI) received unemployment benefits. This was the first-ever scheme in Oman to cover all Omani nationals. Further, by waiving the entitlement conditions, unemployment benefits were given to all Omanis even if they had not been affiliated with the scheme for 12 consecutive months.

The Kuwaiti government continued to pay employment support to existing beneficiaries and provided a six-month unemployment benefit to any citizen suspended from work.

Social Security Contributions

Measures in this area include accepting delayed social security contribution payments and waiving penalties and fees associated with the delays. The Omani government has taken the following measures: (i) postponing the due payments of the monthly contributions (March, April, May, and June 2020) for the employer and employee and (ii) exemption from fines that will result from the delay in paying the due contribution for the months mentioned above only; or resulting from delay in registering their Omani employees/or the notification from the end of their services. In Qatar, the government renewed social security cards that expire from March 15, 2020 until further notice. Beneficiaries of social security include vulnerable categories with no source of income or limited income. The Kuwaiti government postponed the deduction of the replacement part of the retirement pension according to Article (77) of the Law for a period of (six) months. The UAE government postponed the payment of pensions for three months.

Labor Market Measures

The most commonly used labor market instruments across the Gulf countries were labor regulations and shorter work time arrangements (22% of all measures) and were the predominant form of support in the six Gulf countries. Except with Oman and UAE, wage subsidies were widely used labor market instruments adopted by Gulf countries (10% of all measures). In addition, activation measures were adopted only in Saudi and the UAE (4% of all measures) (see Table 2.9).

Table 2.9 Labor market measures, by instruments, by country (number, % of all measures), March 2020–October 2021

	Saudi Arabia	Qatar	Oman	Bahrain	Kuwait	UAE	Total
Activation measures	3 (3%)	0	0	0	0	1 (1%)	4 (4%)
Wage Subsidies	6 (5%)	1 (1%)	0	2 (2%)	2 (2%)	0	10 (10%)
Labor regulations and shorter work time arrangements	6 (5%)	4 (4%)	4 (4%)	3 (3%)	2 (2%)	4 (4%)	23 (22%)

The most common labor market measures adopted by Gulf countries are discussed below.

Wage Subsidies

The Saudi government has supported the full or partial payment of salaries for private-sector workers through the unemployment insurance fund (SANED). The government authorized the use of the unemployment insurance fund to provide support for wage benefits, within certain limits, to private-sector companies who retain their Saudi staff. The government's allocated $80 million for wage support scheme, covering up to 50% of an employee's monthly wage for a period of two years, has supported 133,000 Saudi workers in the private sector (KPMG, 2020). Saudi private-sector workers earning between $853 and $4,000 were eligible for support. The wage support program through SANED has been extended through July 2021, but only to the sectors that are still being affected by COVID-19. In addition, the government allocated $2.4 billion for a furlough scheme to cover 60% of Saudi employees' salaries up to a maximum of $2,400 per employee during three months. Up to 70% of a company's national workforce may be covered for three months (or all of them if the business has five employees or less), provided that the employer can show they have been badly affected by the crisis. Another temporary wage support, the government has subsidized 30%– 50% of the monthly wage of a Saudi employee whose salary ranges from $1,070 to 2,670 for a period of two months. None of the above measures extend to migrant workers.

Moreover, the Saudi government has expanded the coverage of independent workers, which previously did not comply with social insurance legislation, to benefit from wage and employment protection. The government has extended the coverage of COVID-19 relief packages to include food delivery workers, initially excluded from the coronavirus relief packages. Food workers will get the benefits retroactively along with September's 2020 payment. In addition, the government has established a new initiative to support freelancers and those working in the gig economy and provide them with monthly payments of up to $800 for two months. The wage support scheme came in the form of a horizontal expansion of the existing program by extending the coverage of COVID-19 relief packages to include food delivery workers, initially excluded from the coronavirus relief packages. In addition, the government paid the minimum salaries of independent workers in the transportation sector who are registered with the Public Transport Authority but are not under the umbrella of any company, whose activities were affected by the precautionary measures.

In Qatar, the government launched a tiered wage subsidy scheme for six weeks starting March 26, 2020, whereby qualified businesses that experienced a 25% or higher decline in revenues and were not able to continue paying wages were able to get temporary relief. As of May 4, the amount of the subsidy is payable as follows: $400 or 85% of the employee's average net weekly pay, whichever is less, for employees earning less than or equal to $467 per week net; $400 for employees with average net weekly pay between $467 and $567 per week net; $465 or 70% of the employee's average net weekly pay, whichever is less, for employees earning less than or equal to $665 per week net; between $233 and $400 for employees earning between $665 and $1,089 per week net; and less than $400 for employees earning more than $1,089 per week net.

The Bahraini government allocated $572 million for the unemployment insurance fund for 100,000 Bahraini employees working in the private sector for three months. In July 2020, an additional 50% of salaries, for three months, were paid to Bahraini nationals working in the most affected sectors. Lastly, Tamkeen allocated $2.27 million to pay the full salary of kindergarten and nursery employees not insured by the Social Insurance Organization from April to June 2020. In addition, the Tamkeen program allocated $2.27 million to provide $800 to taxi drivers, bus drivers, and driving instructors; and paid the salaries of kindergarten and nursery employees who are not insured by the Social Insurance Organization for three months. Temporary income support was delivered to 400,000 Saudi nationals working in private-sector companies which were affected by the impact of the coronavirus pandemic for May on June 2020. The government disbursed approximately $319 million. This temporary income support covered over 23% of the total number of Saudi nationals in the private sector registered with Saudi Arabia's General Organization for Social Insurance. However, given the uncertainty around the duration of the pandemic, one-off payments are unable to provide recipients with the income security afforded by regular and predictable payments and unlikely to sustainably boost resilience, and are unlikely to enable households to plan for future shocks.

In Kuwait, citizens were paid their monthly salaries for six months starting May 2020, regardless of whether the businesses were closed due to the lockdown with the agreement that the company does not rescind the worker after six months.

Activation Measures

The Saudi government has enacted activation policies to encourage and support jobseekers and other vulnerable groups such as women and people with disabilities to search and find jobs or improve their skills and employability. The government has also adapted and created new programs to train and reskill workers and those entering the labor force during the pandemic and has also allocated the $530 million to support 100,000 job seekers in the private sector (in addition to offering and activating remote work tools as available and alternative options for regular work). In addition, an additional US$400 million has been allocated to add 100,000 new job seekers to the program. A training support track includes US % 213 million to support 100,000 beneficiaries. The government has provided employers 10% additional incentives as long as the maximum support does not exceed 50% of the monthly wage per employee or $800.

UAE

The UAE government implemented distance learning by way of smart mobile apps for all government and private centers for people of determination (disabled) and early intervention centers, in addition to continuing the vocational training project for people of determination to market their products in various outlets.

Labor Regulations and Shorter Work Time Arrangements

Labor regulation adjustments include changes to severance payment obligations, dismissal procedures by easing administrative procedures for the dismissal of migrant workers to facilitate their repatriation, and modifications to leave policies and remuneration to encourage the retention of workers by relaxing labor regulations related to wage reduction and leave policies.

In Saudi Arabia, the government has adjusted its labor market regulations and introduced shorter work time arrangements to retain employment relationships. Together, both policies account for 16% of all labor market policies. Labor regulation adjustments include (i) changes to severance payment obligations by the temporary suspension of the wage protection system (WPS) during early months of the pandemic to ensure that employers can access and continue government services even if wages are delayed or reduced; (ii) dismissal procedures by easing administrative procedures for the dismissal of foreign workers to facilitate their repatriation; and (iii) modifications to leave policies and remuneration to encourage the retention of workers by relaxing labor regulations related to wage reduction and leave policies. The government allowed also changes in employment relationships to lessen the adverse economic impact on businesses arising from the COVID-19 pandemic. These measures include the right to unilaterally decrease salaries by as much as 40% for a period of up to six months, provided that there is a commensurate reduction in working hours. In addition, the government enabled employers to discuss and agree with employees – within six months from the start of the Government-imposed restrictions (i.e., on or about March 16, 2020) (the "COVID-19 Measures Start Date") – three options to lessen the adverse economic impact associated with the work restrictions resulting from the COVID-19 pandemic. These options include (i) reducing the employee's salary commensurate with a reduction in the employee's working hours; (ii) placing the employee on annual leave as a part of his/her annual leave entitlement; and (iii) placing the employee on an exceptional unpaid leave under Article 116 of the Labor Law (ICLG, 2020). The Saudi government also introduced shorter work time arrangements to retain employment relationships. The government has adopted flexible working arrangements for civil servants and private sector workers including options to work from home. In addition, a "flexible work system" targeting private-sector Saudi individuals has been established. The new system allows Saudis to work on an hourly basis while governing the employer-employee relationships in such contractual contexts to reduce labor disputes and enhance performance.

The Omani government allowed private-sector employees in businesses affected by the lockdown to take their paid annual leave during that time. With effect May 2020, the employment contracts of Omani nationals could not be terminated; however, companies facing difficulties due to the lockdowns could make their employees take their annual paid leave after which an employer could negotiate reduced wages and working hours for the following three months. Lastly, employers were required to pay the full salary to employees during the compulsory quarantine period.

The UAE government reduced the fees for obtaining internal work permits and restricted the framework of wages, vacations, and remote working. All focused on the private sector.

Digitalization in Social Protection and Labor Market Responses

Like many other countries (Gentilini et al., 2020), many Gulf countries have relied on the digitization of responses. The Saudi government has introduced a digital platform aimed at promoting and facilitating the hiring from the local market using the "Ajmer portal" (https://www.ajeer.com.sa) which helps foreign workers from being terminated or losing their contractual benefits during the pandemic and also addresses the issue of workers falling into an irregular situation through no fault of their own which, in turn, would reduce the costs and administrative burden of current deportation and amnesty and regularization schemes. This innovative platform has enabled internal labor market mobility. Moreover, an online portal, "Awdah" (https://www.my.gov.sa), was put in place for expatriates' registration wishing to leave the country during the lockdown and COVID pandemic. In addition, the government developed a mobile application called "Sehhaty" (https://sehaty.sa) to register and apply for sick leave. The UAE implemented distance learning by way of smart mobile apps for all government and private centers for people of determination (disabled) and early intervention centers, in addition to continuing the vocational training project for people of determination to market their products in various outlets.

Discussion

This chapter aimed to map social protection and labor market responses to COVID-19 pandemic in six Gulf countries. The study concludes that the Gulf countries conducted a thorough assessment of the circumstances and announced a package of shock-responsive social protection measures totaling 111 measures, building on existing instruments and platforms. Additionally, it demonstrates an overall rapid response via the introduction of (mostly) temporary measures – primarily by relaxing eligibility requirements, increasing benefit levels, and establishing new ad hoc social and job protection schemes. The Gulf states have implemented a mix of new and adapted policies.

As is the case with many high-income countries, Gulf states heavily rely on social assistance and labor market policies to mitigate the pandemic's socio-economic impact. Forty-seven percent of the sample's social protection and labor market policies were social assistance policies, compared to 33% labor market policies and 19% social insurance policies. Saudi Arabia has prioritized labor market policies when it comes to enacting these policies. Kuwait and the UAE were able to expand their social assistance programs. Qatar, Oman, and Bahrain have each implemented a combination of social assistance and labor market policies. This pattern holds when considering various forms of social protection. Saudi Arabia's government has placed a premium on wage subsidies and labor regulations. Kuwait has increased the number of in-kind programs it has implemented. UAE has placed a premium on utility waivers and assistance with financial obligations. Qatar, Oman, and Bahrain have all implemented a combination of labor regulation changes and utility waivers, and financial obligation support. To mitigate the impact of the COVID-19 pandemic and assist vulnerable groups in coping with the shock, Gulf countries have prioritized social assistance measures such as income support and ensuring a minimum level of consumption. Income support for households in the form of exemptions, deferrals, waivers of utility payments, rent assistance, and financial obligations was the most common type of social assistance in the Gulf region. Except for Kuwait, all Gulf countries have placed a premium on assisting citizens and migrants with household income support. Additionally, while nearly half of SP measures targeted only citizens, there is a trend toward providing universal support to all affected individuals.

Cash transfers intended to supplement income have been used less frequently. Gulf countries have implemented new emergency cash transfers, repurposed existing ones, or expanded existing ones to include new beneficiaries and/or increase benefit values. Certain countries expanded their programs vertically by supplementing payments to existing beneficiaries. Others have expanded social assurance programs horizontally by increasing the number of beneficiaries of existing cash transfer programs, establishing temporary emergency cash transfer schemes, or focusing emergency cash transfers on vulnerable population groups (e.g., female-headed- households, widows or pregnant women, elderly people, households with children or orphans, people with disabilities). However, cash transfer programs remain inaccessible to the majority of migrant workers, and the rules governing formal access for these groups have remained unchanged throughout the pandemic. Another way of ensuring minimum consumption is for Gulf countries to provide in-kind transfers to those in need, primarily in the form of food, food baskets, and sanitation materials for vulnerable families, as well as Ramadan-related food transfers.

To stabilize the demand for migrant workers and increase labor market efficiency (Betcherman, 2015; Devarajan et al., 1997), Gulf countries prioritized labor regulation changes such as increased job flexibility, job rotations, shorter working hours, or other flexible work arrangements, changing remuneration policies, and requiring employers to pay to leave for private-sector workers, including in the case of self-quarantine or granting a special license. Additionally, Gulf countries have permitted new working conditions, regulating wage reduction, dismissal procedures, hiring flexibility, and leave policies that were not previously spelled out in law. Additionally, governments have amended labor regulations to strengthen health and workplace safety requirements. These regulations vary significantly across Gulf countries, with some prohibiting firms from terminating employees (primarily citizens), while others allow them to temporarily cancel employee contracts. Similarly, some countries permitted firms to reduce compensation, while others required increased allowances for citizens.

To safeguard jobs and support labor income and the unemployed, Gulf countries have placed a premium on labor supply policies such as wage subsidies, unemployment benefits, and training and placement assistance (activation measures). Labor income support policies, such as unemployment benefits and wage subsidies, have been less widely used to increase workers' and unemployed workers' disposable income. Gulf countries prioritized wage subsidies accompanied by unemployment benefits to assist private-sector workers in receiving their salaries in full or in part. Nonetheless, labor income support and activation measures remain inaccessible to the majority of migrant workers, and the rules governing formal access to these benefits have remained unchanged throughout the pandemic. To compensate for these groups' income losses, Gulf countries proposed a variety of temporary (and occasionally one-off) measures, most notably changes to labor regulations or delivery modality, waivers of conditionality, and flexibilization of payment duties.

Throughout the Gulf region, social insurance measures have been less prevalent. Additionally, each country has implemented at least one social insurance policy. Paid leave and health insurance to ensure access to free treatment and testing, including for those who were not insured, were the most widely used forms of social insurance. Social contribution measures such as reducing or deferring employer and employee contributions, adjusting social security benefits such as pensions, and increasing pensions or providing one-time benefits to social insurance system retirees have been less common. The majority of social insurance policies have been designed exclusively to benefit citizens.

Special Measures to Support Migrant Workers

At the outbreak of the pandemic, the cramped labor camps that house the majority of low-wage migrant workers in Gulf countries became breeding grounds for COVID-19 and were forced to be isolated with entry and exit restricted (Equidem, 2020). As the months passed, the Saudi economy contracted as a result of lockdowns and other measures imposed to contain the spread of Covid-19, as well as the pandemic-induced precipitous decline in global oil prices, resulting in layoffs, pay cuts, payment delays, and other financial difficulties for migrants of all skill levels (Ekanayake, 2020). Migrants were discovered to be one of the most vulnerable groups in Saudi Arabia during this lockdown, as their very livelihoods came to a halt, as did their family's status in the origin country. Numerous migrant workers face unemployment or income reduction, are stranded in the country with little or no assistance, and are unable to support their families at home (Equidem, 2020). As a result, Gulf countries have taken steps to ensure that migrant workers, including those in an irregular situation, have access to basic health and social assistance services, including free testing and treatment (Saudi Arabia, Qatar), ensuring that foreign workers receive their full salaries, even while in quarantine (Qatar), providing food transfers to those in need, including foreign workers (Saudi Arabia, Oman, Kuwait), and exempting foreign workers who become irregular from taxation (Saudi Arabia, Oman (UAE).

Conclusion

The Gulf countries' social protection and labor market responses to COVID-19 provide ample learning opportunities. Given the imperative of providing emergency assistance to those in need (e.g., migrant workers, who are frequently excluded from social protection), Gulf countries were forced to be innovative in their approach to social protection and labor market measures. Gulf countries have been forced to adopt technological innovations and revise their social protection administrative processes. Given that the crisis's consequences will entail significant job losses and increased vulnerability in Gulf countries over the medium term, the need for innovative and sustainable SP practices becomes even more apparent. Additionally, the COVID-19 crisis exposed critical coverage gaps among a large number of migrant workers who were disproportionately impacted by government policies. Due to their lack of social insurance coverage and their poverty, those migrant workers are particularly vulnerable during times of hardship. The lack of financial support for migrant workers, as well as wage reductions, payment delays, and non-payment, raises concerns about abusive working conditions and forced labor, especially for migrant workers who are in debt due to exploitative recruitment fees and the kafala system's forced dependency. Thus, comprehensive social protection strategies that incorporate migrant workers into national social protection responses are consistent with international human rights, international labor standards, and the International Labour Organization's Centenary Declaration for the Future of Work and are founded on the principles of equality of treatment and non-discrimination, which will be critical in mitigating the effects of COVID-19 and promoting a faster recovery (ILO, 2020b). Expanding the social insurance system to include migrant workers could be a critical component of Gulf countries' social protection policies. This is critical if the Gulf region is to weather current and future crises. In the longer term, it is necessary to pursue effective structural transformation, legislative and policy reforms, including a universal safety net and welfare innovation.

The COVID-19 pandemic has also created employment opportunities throughout the Gulf region. As a result of the economic slowdown, a large number of migrant workers are returning to their home countries, creating a massive void that can easily be filled by citizens, as the majority of Gulf countries have already implemented nationalization programs that require expatriate workers to be gradually replaced by a local workforce. However, local workers' skill levels must be rapidly upgraded to meet labor market demands.

References

Alamri, H. S., Algarni, A., Shehata, S. F., Al Bshabshe, A., Alshehri, N. N., ALAsiri, A. M., Hussain, A. H., Alalmay, A. Y., Alshehri, E. A., Alqarni, Y., & Saleh, N. F. (2020). Prevalence of depression, anxiety, and stress among the general population in Saudi Arabia during the COVID-19 pandemic. *International Journal of Environmental Research and Public Health*, *17*(24), 9183. https://doi.org/10.3390/ijerph17249183

Alenazi, T. H., BinDhim, N. F., Alenazi, M. H., Tamim, H., Almagrabi, R. S., Aljohani, S. M., H Basyouni, M., Almubark, R. A., Althumiri, N. A., & Alqahtani, S. A. (2020). Prevalence and predictors of anxiety among healthcare workers in Saudi Arabia during the COVID-19 pandemic. *Journal of Infection and Public Health*, *13*(11), 1645–1651. https://doi.org/10.1016/j.jiph.2020.09.001

Algahtani, F. D., Hassan, S., Alsaif, B., & Zrieq, R. (2021). Assessment of the quality of life during COVID-19 pandemic: A cross-sectional survey from the Kingdom of Saudi Arabia. *International Journal of Environmental Research and Public Health*, *18*(3), 847. https://doi.org/10.3390/ijerph18030847

Alkhamees, A. A., Alrashed, S. A., Alzunaydi, A. A., Almohimeed, A. S., & Aljohani, M. S. (2020). The psychological impact of the COVID-19 pandemic on the general population of Saudi Arabia. *Comprehensive Psychiatry*, *102*, 152192. https://doi.org/10.1016/j.comppsych.2020.152192

Alshehri, F. S., Alatawi, Y., Alghamdi, B. S., Alhifany, A. A., & Alharbi, A. (2020). Prevalence of post-traumatic stress disorder during the COVID-19 pandemic in Saudi Arabia. *Saudi Pharmaceutical Journal*, *28*(12), 1666–1673. https://doi.org/10.1016/j.jsps.2020.10.013

Alyami, M. H., Naser, A. Y., Orabi, M. A., Alwafi, H., & Alyami, H. S. (2020). Epidemiology of COVID-19 in the Kingdom of Saudi Arabia: An ecological study. *Frontiers in Public Health*, 8. https://doi.org/10.3389/fpubh.2020.00506

Alyoubi, A., Halstead, E. J., Zambelli, Z., & Dimitriou, D. (2021). The impact of the COVID-19 pandemic on students' mental health and sleep in Saudi Arabia. *International Journal of Environmental Research and Public Health*, *18*(17), 9344. https://doi.org/10.3390/ijerph18179344

Balkhi, F., Nasir, A., Zehra, A., & Riaz, R. (2020). Psychological and behavioral response to the coronavirus (COVID-19) pandemic. *Cureus 12*(5). https://doi.org/10.7759/cureus.7923

Bastagli, F. (2014). *Responding to a crisis: The design and delivery of social protection* (vol. 90). ODI, London, UK. https://cdn.odi.org/media/documents/9040.pdf

Bastagli, F., & Lowe, C. (2021). *Social protection response to Covid-19 and beyond Emerging evidence and learning for future crises* (Working Paper 614). ODI, London, UK. https://cdn.odi.org/media/documents/ODI_Synthesis_2010_4GfT5Rv.pdf

Betcherman, G. (2014). Labor market regulations: What do we know about their impacts in developing countries? *The World Bank Research Observer*, *30*(1), 124–153. https://doi.org/10.1093/wbro/lku005

Devarajan, S., Squire, L., & Suthiwart-Narueput, S. (1997). Beyond rate of return: Reorienting project appraisal. *The World Bank Research Observer*, *12*(1), 35–46. https://doi.org/10.1093/wbro/12.1.35

Devereux, S. (2021). Social protection responses to COVID-19 in Africa. *Global Social Policy*, *21*(3), 421–447. https://doi.org/10.1177/14680181211021260

Ekanayake, A. (2020). *Covid-19 pandemic and the labour migrants in the Gulf corporation council (GCC) region*. The Migrant.

El Keshky, M. E., Alsabban, A. M., & Basyouni, S. S. (2021). The psychological and social impacts on personal stress for residents quarantined for COVID-19 in Saudi Arabia. *Archives of Psychiatric Nursing*, *35*(3), 311–316. https://doi.org/10.1016/j.apnu.2020.09.008

Equidem. (2020). *The Cost of Contagion: The human rights impacts of COVID-19 on migrant workers in the Gulf*. Equidem, London, UK. https://www.equidem.org/assets/downloads/1837_Equidem_The_Cost_of_Congation_Report_ART_WEB.pdf

Gentilini, U., Almenfi, M., & Dale, P. (2020). *Social protection and jobs responses to COVID-19: A real-time review of country measures* ("Living paper" version 14). https://documents1.worldbank.org/curated/en/467521607723220511/pdf/Social-Protection-and-Jobs-Responses-to-COVID-19-A-Real-Time-Review-of-Country-Measures-December-11-2020.pdf

Grosh, M., Fruttero, A., & Oliveri, M. L. (2013). *Understanding the poverty impact of the global financial crisis in Latin America and the Caribbean – Part II: The role of social protection'* [Paper presentation]. IZA conference, Washington, DC: World Bank.

ICLG. (2020). *Employment & labour law 2021 in Saudi Arabia.* International Comparative Legal Guides International Business Reports. Global Legal Group, London, UK. https://iclg.com/practice-areas/employment-and-labour-laws-and-regulations/saudi-arabia

ILO. (2020a). *Social protection responses to the COVID-19 crisis in the MENA/Arab States region.* https://www.ilo.org/wcmsp5/groups/public/—arabstates/—ro-beirut/documents/publication/wcms_756764.pdf

ILO. (2020b). *Social protection for migrant workers: A necessary response to the Covid-19 crisis* (ILO brief, June 2020). https://www.ilo.org/wcmsp5/groups/public/—ed_protect/—soc_sec/documents/publication/wcms_748979.pdf

Iqbal, S. A., & Tayyab, N. (2020). COVID-19 and children: The mental and physical reverberations of the pandemic. *Child: Care, Health and Development, 47*(1), 136–139. https://doi.org/10.1111/cch.12822

KPMG. (2020). *Saudi Arabia Budget Report 2021.* Dammam, Kingdom of Saudi Arabia. https://assets.kpmg/content/dam/kpmg/sa/pdf/2020/kpmg-saudi-arabia-budget-report-2021.pdf

Sonbol, H., Alahdal, H. M., Alanazi, R. A., Alsamhary, K., & Ameen, F. (2021). COVID-19 pandemic causing depression in different Sociodemographic groups in Saudi Arabia. *International Journal of Environmental Research and Public Health, 18*(13), 6955. https://doi.org/10.3390/ijerph18136955

Worldmeters.info. (2020, November 30). *Coronavirus Cases.* Worldometer. https://www.worldometers.info

3 Small GCC States' Responses to COVID-19

The UAE and Qatar

Diana Galeeva

Introduction

Large states with significant populations and territory, such as the US, India, Brazil and Russia, are standardly regarded as particularly influential within realist International Relations (IR) theory. However, they have proven to be among the most challenged by the COVID-19 outbreak, struggling to deal with the pandemic and suffering ever-growing human and economic losses. In contrast, some small states with corresponding geographical area and population, but with a strong economy and high state capacity, appear to have the ability to successfully address their national security concerns caused by the pandemic. They have even, surprisingly, been able to diversify their financial resources by providing foreign aid globally. Why have some small GCC states, such as the UAE and Qatar, been better able to maintain their national security and at the same time have a global reach during such globally insecure times?

The differential impact of COVID-19 raises questions about the neo-realist tradition which considers small territories with small populations as 'weak'. During this global pandemic, such small countries can be 'strong', if the situation leads to economic advantages. For example, due to their small populations, the UAE and Qatar have been able to distribute their resources and protect citizens from the pandemic. These advantages are related to high state capacity and control by its leadership over their citizens, borders and territory, as a result of total surveillance and resources. At the same time, the UAE and Qatar have provided significant foreign aid, a litmus test of influence in world politics. An alternative IR literature which focuses on small states and alternative sources of power is more helpful for understanding these small state states' foreign aid initiatives as an effective response to the pandemic. Overall, the pandemic – through the lens of foreign aid – has underlined the emergence of small GCC states on the global stage as potentially 'strong' states. This chapter will examine the neo-realist stance by positioning it within the COVID-19 pandemic literature. It will then offer an examination of neo-realist literature in the context of small Gulf states, followed by discussion of the UAE and Qatar responses to the pandemic.

DOI: 10.4324/9781003266259-3

Finally, the chapter will present the implications for policy and practice, relevant limitations and directions of future research and broader conclusions.

Neo-Realist Literature in the Age of COVID-19

The pandemic challenges the existing literature concerning the neo-realist tradition, which posits that only great powers can be influential, while small states' limited capacities render them vulnerable. This neo-realist 'power resources' approach measures the tangible resources of states, including their military strength, their size of population and territory, resource endowment, economic capacity, political stability and competence (Waltz, 1979). However, the pandemic has demonstrated that the so-called 'great powers' can in certain circumstances be quite vulnerable because of the greater possibility of the spread of a pandemic: the difficulty in controlling the spread because the systems and population distribution are necessarily more complex in a bigger country. By contrast, a small state with a small population but high resources of wealth can allow an astute government to apply more flexible measures. For example, a large percentage of the population could be tested, social-distancing/isolation measures would be more easily enforced, and the healthcare system could cope with the relatively small number of cases who would need to be hospitalized.

Neo-realists see the fear of anarchy as a key cause of competition for security and therefore such threats, such as an armed confrontation, would normally emerge from other states. In contrast, COVID-19 is an invisible 'enemy' from a national security perspective. Some recent attempts to theorize about the coronavirus crisis suggest a focus on the Securitization concept, which is associated with the Copenhagen School of security studies. Hoffman (2020) proposes to 'securitize' COVID-19 as a global health issue and as a threat to national security. He stresses the language of battle and war used by global leaders to show the challenge posed by the coronavirus. However, COVID-19 is a human security global threat, rather than an inter-state military one. Consequently, it can be argued that foreign aid rather than military aid becomes relatively more significant in terms of consolidating alliances. In other words, because of their state capacity and economic strength, small GCC states have been able to join other 'strong' and 'weak' states in providing foreign aid to deal with this invisible 'enemy' globally, thus demonstrating that the neo-realists' traditional arguments explaining domestic and international policies appear to be no longer adequate.

Neo-Realist Literature in the Context of Small GCC States

An absolute power approach, based on quantitative criteria, is part of the neo-realist tradition which considers small states as 'weak powers', more preoccupied with survival than great powers and without real power in international relations (Keohane, 1969; Elman, 1995). This absolute definition is a sign of 'size', that is, area, armed capacity, population and GNP (Masaryk, 1966; Vital, 1967; Keohane, 1969). Micro-states have been understood as states with populations of less than 1 million (Clarke and Payne, 1987). In the context of the neo-realist tradition, the small Gulf states are in possession of one indicator of power. The UAE's GDP was worth USD 425 bn in 2019, while GDP per capita was 40,782.40. In 2019, Qatar's GDP was worth USD 201bn, some 0.17% of the world economy (Trading Economics, 2019). However, applying other indicators of the neo-realist schools' assessment, the small GCC states' capacity to demonstrate power is limited. The UAE's territory of 77,700 km^2 contains a population of 10 million people, of which only 11.48% are Emiratis. Qatar is only 11,437 sq. km (4,247 sq. miles) in area (Fromherz, 2012). In 2020, Qatar's population totalled 2,874,381, so if applying an approach based solely on quantitative criteria, it is also defined as a small state. However, with only approximately 300,000 of the population deemed to be Qatari citizens (Wright, 2016), Qatar is, perhaps, a micro-state.

At the same time, due to strong economic capacity and small populations, the small GCC states are among the richest in the world. At the regional level, the Arab Spring 2011 was particularly crucial for taking advantage of such state characteristics, and their political influence soared due to their available wealth for use in active foreign policies. Added to this, the regional architecture, namely the transformed geopolitical balance of power in the Middle East and North African (MENA) region, the shift in US foreign policy towards Asia and fears of the local effect of the Arab uprising in the GCC states, spread small GCC states' political influence within the Middle East (Watanabe, 2017; Young, 2019). The power vacuum in the Middle East entailed a decreasing role for traditional leaders – Iraq, Egypt and Syria – and promoted the leadership opportunities of the GCC states. The GCC states, in particular Saudi Arabia, the UAE and Qatar, have been the most dominant in the Middle East since 2011. The changing political environment and active position of the GCC states have led to attempts to revise and clarify the terms 'weak' and 'strong' in studies of the region (Kamrava, 2016) and placing 'small' GCC states among the region's political players. In other words, the regional architecture created in the context of the Arab Spring contributed to a challenge to neo-realist perspectives of 'small' and 'strong' states. Within almost ten years, this combination of states' characteristics has become essential to address the challenges posed by COVID-19, as well as important in understanding the spread of international leverage by offering foreign aid, as will be illustrated below.

Empirical Findings: The UAE and Qatar Responses to COVID-19

The UAE and Qatar Responses to COVID-19: At the National Level

Due to the UAE's small population, it has proven easier to limit the spread of COVID-19 than in many other countries. By 7 December 2020, the UAE had recorded 177,577 cases and 594 deaths (Worldometers, 2020a). A variety of measures had been taken in March and April to protect its citizens. Within a month (by April 26), 14 drive-through test centres had been established, with free daily screening for 10,000 essential workers, a testing laboratory having been built within a fortnight. By 25 May 2020, UAE officials announced that more than 2m people had been tested, suggesting that widespread and accessible testing had become a priority for the UAE and the key to curbing the spread of the virus.

Each emirate within the UAE tackled the pandemic somewhat differently. In Dubai's case, this was strongly influenced by economic factors, specifically the desire to maintain a strong economy post-coronavirus. The pandemic definitely challenged the 'Dubai model', which is a key regional trade and transport hub which developed in the 1990s: the spread of the virus caused airlines to shut down, stifled global trade and foreign investment and hit tourism, cultural linkages and exchanges (Gray, 2011). Dubai became the first to ease lockdown measures in order to preserve its status as a 'business hub'. At the beginning of Ramadan, retailers who normally expect to cater for a rush of shoppers were allowed to open and individuals were allowed to leave their homes between 6 a.m. and 10 p.m. without a permit. Dubai's malls, cafes and restaurants were reopened under strict conditions, including limiting the number of visitors to 30% capacity, maintaining social distancing and wearing masks (Fattah, 2020).

On 26 April, Dubai Roads and Transport Authority confirmed that the emirate was resuming its metro, taxi services and public buses (Naar, 2020a). From 30 May, businesses reopened, including gyms, fitness clubs, sports academies and cinemas with continued social distancing and regular disinfection. Shopping malls were fully opened, as well as all other private sector businesses. Additionally, the Supreme Committee of Crisis and Disaster Management announced that Dubai welcomed tourists from 7 July 2020, on condition of presenting a recent COVID-19 negative certificate (Government of Dubai Media Office, 2020). In order to maintain the successful 'Dubai model' and attract more tourists, it has begun to brand itself as one of safest destinations. Dubai authorities have launched different initiatives, including a suggested 'DUBAI ASSURED' stamp, a compliance programme to acknowledge and certify retail and tourism establishments that fit with all public health protocols for the management and prevention of COVID-19 (Naar, 2020b).

Asad Aburumman of the University of Sharjah (2020) argues that despite Dubai's tourism sector's announcements about reopening, 'people worldwide were still afraid of travelling. Consequently, the numbers of international arrivals in Dubai were far from those before March 2020'. Such an outcome was almost inevitable because of the existing measures and the wider challenges of COVID-19, such as social distancing, self-isolation, travel restrictions and lack of vaccine. Importantly, international bans affected more than 90% of the global population and included widespread restrictions on tourism and community mobility (Gössling et al., 2020). This suggests that globalisation, which was the key to many successful economy diversifications pre-pandemic, instead creates challenges in such uncertain times (even leaving aside its role in the spread of the virus). In other words, because the 'Dubai model' relies heavily on globalisation, it was heavily hit by the pandemic, and attempts to bringing some tourism in July could not fully deal with the core of the problem. Ultimately, the pandemic is a 'human threat' (rather than a military one, which the neo-realist tradition focuses on). The 'Dubai model' has proven to be successful pre-pandemic but requires further re-consideration in such uncertain times, especially within the context of the predicted recession and global financial crisis, as further outcomes of COVID-19 (IMF, 2020).

Other emirates took quite a different approach, taking a long time to ease the lockdown. Abu Dhabi, whose wealth relies mainly on massive oil and gas reserves, as well as its importance as the capital and political centre of the UAE, announced new regulations via the Supreme Council for National Security and the Department of Health. As a result, private beaches at hotels were reopened on 1 June with a reduced capacity and social-distancing measures (Shirka, 2020). As of 14 June, dog walkers, cyclists and walkers were allowed to return to Abu Dhabi's Corniche as part of the UAE's easing of restrictions, reopening of pools, gyms and hotels. However, restrictions on entering and exiting Abu Dhabi were prolonged 'as the government carries out a major testing drive in densely populated areas of the capital' (Ryan, 2020). It was only on 4 July that officials in Abu Dhabi eased travel restrictions for residents, allowing short trips outside of the emirate, on provision of a negative COVID-19 test (GardaWorld, 2020). On 28 May, Ras Al Khaimah, a less wealthy emirate, reopened shopping malls and public beaches, while gyms, cinemas, entertainment venues and common seating areas, along with prayer rooms within malls, remained closed (Haza, 2020).

The UAE's strong oil-based economy was also challenged by a substantial drop in oil prices caused by Saudi's response to Moscow's refusal to reduce oil production in March 2020. Moscow's determination to sustain working relations amid such disagreements became visible by October. Brent crude has been trading between USD 40 and USD 45 since July, capped by the impact of the coronavirus outbreak on global energy demand, though supported by the OPEC+ production cut (Blas and Arkhipov, 2020). Despite such challenges, based on IMF predictions, the UAE's economy is expected to decline by 3.5% in 2020. These are better indicators in comparison to the fall in real GDP of most other energy-based economies: Saudi Arabia (6.8%), Qatar (4.3%), Bahrain (3.6%), Oman (2.8%) and Kuwait (1.1%).

Retaining economic strength and protecting the already small population will be further important for dealing with the pandemic. By the middle of January 2021, the UAE has already become second behind Israel globally, having 11.8 doses of the vaccine per 100 people. This initiative is in line with UAE's plan to vaccinate more than 50% of the country's population (Khaleej Times, 2021). The UAE offers available vaccines from around the globe to its citizens: in December 2020, Dubai began inoculating people with the COVID-19 vaccine produced by Pfizer and BioNTec. Abu Dhabi began Phase III clinical trials of Russia's experimental COVID-19 vaccine, known as Sputnik V in early 2021. The UAE has already been conducting Phase III trials of a COVID-19 vaccine developed by the China National Pharmaceutical Group (Sinopharm) (Al-Arabiya, 2021). Despite challenges facing the world, the UAE has tackled the pandemic comparatively successfully (so far), and this has been especially beneficial to its foreign policies during the pandemic, as will be demonstrated after an examination of Qatar's domestic response to the pandemic.

In Qatar, there were 141,272 total cases and 241 deaths by 15 December 2020 (Worldometers, 2020b). The virus mainly arrived in Qatar carried by nationals returning from Iran. The first reported case was a Qatari national who had been in Iran. Additionally, cases increased as employers in the central market and a hypermarket tested positive. As a result, all schools and universities were closed, mosques were closed and Friday prayers suspended, while speedy tracing and testing were implemented. Qatar's small population was rather advantageous in all this process, and this resulted in low death rates. For example, based on Johns Hopkins University figures, in Qatar, it was 0.3%, in Kuwait – 0.1%, in Bahrain – 0.6% and in Saudi Arabia – 1.4% (Jones, 2020). Marc Jones (2020) of Hamad bin Khalifa University explains that 'most Gulf countries have demographic characteristics with a relatively small elderly population ... as Covid-19 is more deadly to those aged 70 and above, this could partly explain why Qatar has a relatively low mortality rate'. However, as these figures demonstrate, even at the beginning of COVID-19 outbreak by the beginning of March, it can be observed that the Gulf states with smaller populations had fewer positive cases in total, in comparison to Saudi Arabia, which is the most populous GCC member.

Moreover, the small population of Qatar contributed to the lowest death rate, alongside Qatar's wealth advantages, because it made it possible to conduct extensive testing and allowed significant healthcare spending (Al-Jazeera, 2020a). For example, reportedly, by 20 May, two field hospitals were opened in Qatar in just two weeks (GHD, 2020). In one month, it was reported that five hospitals had been designed, four testing centres and an isolation hospital for COVID-19 cases were established (The Peninsula, 2020). Current global challenges of COVID-19 and the crash of oil prices in 2020 have also affected the economy, based on the prediction of the World Bank that Qatar's growth is to stall, even with its policy to raise government spending to ease the economic implications of COVID-19, and its aim for 3% growth in the medium term, driven by stronger activity in the service sector, such as the FIFA World Cup 2022, underpinning a V-shaped recovery. Thus, Qatar's wealth factor remains central to fighting the virus, and despite negative predictions of the impact of the pandemic, it is resilient in the face of continuing challenges, mainly due to its energy revenues. This has also assisted it in providing foreign aid to other states, as will be further examined below.

Foreign Aid by the UAE and Qatar During the COVID-19

The UAE's policies in fighting the pandemic can be seen as a savvy attempt to increase its influence, pursuing a cooperative strategy, which has included making alliances. The UAE's economic strength, combined with the small number of cases of COVID-19 domestically, has allowed it to emerge, remarkably, as the world's largest aid donor during the pandemic. By the middle of December 2020, the UAE humanitarian aid had surpassed 1.675 tons and helped 1.6m medical workers globally. By comparison, by the half of the year (January–July), the UAE had already delivered 1.087 tons to 73 nations, supported 1m medical workers worldwide.

Although the UAE has been acknowledged as the largest Arab aid donor since the 1970s, its humanitarian aid programme during the pandemic has taken a leap forward. Prior to that, the UAE provided aid mostly to poorer Arab and Muslim countries (Al Mezaini, 2012). During the COVID-19 pandemic, it continued to distribute foreign aid to Muslim populated countries and territories and expanded its help to other territories where Muslims are inhabitants. For example, it has sent aid to Russian Muslim regions (Chechnya and Dagestan) and areas in Central Asia states. In 2009, it provided foreign aid only to Kazakhstan (Al Mezaini, 2012); however, since the pandemic started, it has sent aid to Tajikistan, Uzbekistan, Kyrgyzstan and Kazakhstan. This is no coincidence, as in recent years it has boosted its bilateral relations with the Central Asian states (Ismail, 2020). With regard to relations with Russian Muslim regions, the UAE has been developing close cooperation with most of them, particularly since the early 2000s, especially with the Chechen Republic, whose head, Ramzan Kadyrov even addressed Mohammad bin Zayed, as a 'brother' (Galeeva, 2020).

The UAE's foreign aid programme during the pandemic has thus demonstrated its global reach. It has donated aid throughout Africa (Mauritania, Madagascar, The Democratic Republic of Congo, Sudan, Gambia, Somalia, Sierra Leone, Niger, Mali, Zimbabwe, Guinea, Kenya, Botswana, South Africa, Ethiopia, among others); Asia (Philippines, Afghanistan, Bangladesh, India, Maldives, Nepal, Pakistan, Kazakhstan, Kyrgyzstan, among others); South America (Chile, Uruguay, Peru, Colombia, among others); North America (Costa Rica, Dominican Republic, among others) and Europe (Croatia, Greece, Cyprus, Romania, Italy, among others). Remarkably, it provided foreign aid to EU members, particularly when some prioritized their own national needs over others (Braw, 2020). Moreover, as with previous humanitarian aid efforts, the UAE provided aid to some Eastern European states, such as Ukraine and Belarus and in the South Caucasus, including Armenia and Azerbaijan. Therefore, in contrast to previous initiatives, the UAE provided aid to all types, 'weak' and 'strong' states.

This extensive foreign aid programme has enabled the UAE to emerge as the world's largest aid donor during the pandemic, alongside other 'strong' states. China, for example, where the centre of the outbreak began, had provided aid to over 130 counties and international organizations by the 10 April (CGTN, 2020), while the US provided USD 274m of emergency health, disaster and humanitarian aid by March 31 (Reynold, 2020). Some other small states with a high economic capacity have also managed the outbreak effectively (so far) but have not been as generous as the UAE on the foreign aid front. As reported on 26 March 2020, Norway (a well-known aid donor) contributed approximately USD 1,045,445.00 in humanitarian aid in response to the pandemic. It also contributed USD 1,568,617.50 as its portion of the UN Central Emergency Response Fund. An additional USD 9,411,705.00 supported the implementation of the UN Global Humanitarian Response Plan to the pandemic. Rather than supporting particular states, Norway prefers to support world organizations, such as the UN, Norwegian humanitarian organizations and the International Red Cross and Red Crescent movement (Reliefweb, 2020).

Another notable Arab donor, Qatar, also provided foreign aid to different states worldwide. According to the International Cooperation Department Ministry of Foreign Affairs report (2020) on Qatar's aid to friendly countries to confront the emerging coronavirus, as of August 2020, Qatar had offered about USD 50m in foreign aid to 32 countries, through the Ministry of Defence, the Ministry of Foreign Affairs and the Qatar Fund for Development. International organisations, civil societies and humanitarian associations also provided USD 20m to the Global Alliance for Vaccines and Immunization (GAVI) to speed up research on testing, assisting the development of the vaccine and medication. Qatar also offered USD 10m to the World Health Organisation, to assist with swift access, to offer equipment for the test, and the provision of adequate vaccine. Aid receipts are located mainly in the MENA region (Jordan, Lebanon, Palestine, Tunisia, Algeria, Sudan, Somalia, Iran, Iraq), but Qatar also offered help to 'strong' states, such as the USA, China, and members of the European Union (Italy, France, Spain).

Foreign aid during COVID-19 by Qatar might suggest continuation of its policies. For example, the Ministry of Defence offered USD 150m to the Gaza Strip, in order to support the health sector, to fight COVID-19 locally. On 23 October 2012, Qatar's leadership were the first Arab leaders to visit Gaza since Hamas assumed power in 2007 (Ulrichsen, 2014). The former amir, Shayk Hamad pledged more Qatari investment (from USD 250m to USD 400m) for urgently needed health, housing and infrastructural projects in Gaza (Rudoren, 2012). Moreover, in November 2018, Israel allowed Qatar to start a six-month cash infusion of USD 90m into Gaza for civil service wages and fuel, but a third cash donation of USD 15m in January 2019 was blocked due to violence on the border (The Jerusalem Post, 2019). The former Israeli defence minister said that Qatari payments are 'the continuation of the process of surrendering to terrorists and Hamas' (ibid). The Qatar Foreign Minister, Mohammad bin 'Abdulrahman al-Thani, stated in his speech at the Munich Security Conference in 2019 (Amer, 2019) that Qatari support for Gaza would continue, and denied that it funds groups that are labelled terrorists, including Hamas, but was rather 'trying to put an end to the humanitarian crisis in Gaza'. Reports from May 2019 support this speech, as the Qatari foreign minister revealed plans to send USD 480m to help Palestinians in the West Bank and Gaza (*The Guardian*, 2019). In other words, foreign aid connected to COVID-19 to the Gaza Strip continues Qatar's policies in the region.

Non-governmental aid also occurred through institutions, charitable organisations and private sector companies of Qatar, and almost USD 30m in donations to 66 countries. These included relief, medical and financial support, and the aid was offered via its offices across the globe by Qatar Red Crescent, Qatar Charity, Al Majida Group, 'Baladna Food Industries' Qatar National Bank and Qatar Airways. As the report of the Ministry of Foreign Affairs says, Qatar Airways played a key role in delivering foreign aid and was vital to transporting 1 million people across the globe and managing to fly them safely. Neither the role of charitable organisations nor that of Qatar Airways is accidental or should be surprising in view of Qatar's foreign policies, especially for its state-branding.

For example, in 2011, the charitable entity the Qatar Foundation for Education, Science and Community, also known as the Qatar Foundation (QF), paid EUR 150m (USD 168 m) for a five-year deal to become FC Barcelona's first ever shirt sponsor. Likewise, Qatar Airways was the main sponsor of FC Barcelona between 2011 and 2017, following a EUR 96 m (USD 107m) deal (Conn, 2017). In 2011, the airline initially signed a five-year deal with Barcelona for EUR 215 m (USD 241m) and extended it another year in 2017 (Dillon, 2018). Qatar Airways also acted as an official partner of the cycling Tour of Qatar and Qatar Open Tennis Tournament in 2011, was the title sponsor of the EuroHockey Nations Championships in 2007 and was the official airline for English Test Cricket and Formula E motor racing (Garcia and Amara, 2013:11).

Qatar Airways signed a five-year partnership agreement with FC Bayern Munich to become its 'platinum partner' until June 2023 (Dillon, 2018). The airline took over the sponsorship contract that Bayern had signed with Hamad International Airport (HIA) in 2016 and extended it to include a sleeve sponsorship in 2017. HIA's sponsorship arrangement with Bayern was estimated to cost at least EUR 10m (USD 11m) and has been even more profitable for the Bavarian team. Both Hamad International Airport and Qatar Airways are state-owned. Another example was Qatar Airways' announcement on 23 April 2018 of a multi-year collaboration agreement with the Italian football club, AS Roma. This was the largest deal ever signed by the club and it ensured that Qatar Airways would become Roma's main worldwide partner, with the airline's logo adorning the team's shirts through the 2020–2021 season (Roma, 2018). As Qatar's example illustrates, it continued policies of offering foreign aid, including the involvement of governmental institutions in collaboration with charitable organisations and the private sector.

Implications for Policy and Practice

The small size of both (economically strong) states, the UAE and Qatar, have been shown to make it easier to control the spread of the virus. At the national level, in dealing with the pandemic, the 'vulnerabilities' of a small state can turn out to be advantageous because by closing its borders, and with a relatively small number of citizens to manage, its national security concerns prompted by the virus are minimal. Moreover, considering the pandemic as a human interaction threat, rather than an inter-military one, a state's economic strength can be viewed as central to the development of policies designed to increase that state's global influence. For these reasons, this chapter is a call to review and perhaps develop further the IR literature, particularly with regard to the measurement of the power of states during such unprecedented times and into an uncertain future.

At the policymaking level, the impact on a state's security of the first wave of the pandemic can be measured as follows. Policymakers are being required to project speedy and new policies in order to tackle security challenges effectively; policies that do not seem to fit any existing models of the International Relations theory or Political Science. At the national level, the pandemic demonstrates the crucial importance to any country of being able to provide advanced health assistance to its all citizens at any time. Moreover, globalisation has emerged arguably as a negative factor, because the pandemic is a human interaction threat, which has helped to further spread the virus. At the same, as the 'Dubai model' suggests, relying on globalisation to diversify the economy during a pandemic is also problematic. This might be considered while further developing strategies and forecasting possible scenarios of post-pandemic economic recovery. Already there are important research and suggestions by international organisations (IMF, 2020) and UAE scholars (Alshamsi, 2020) worth consideration. This can be considered while further developing national programmes, such as the UAE Centennial 2071 – a long-term, full-vision plan – map of the long-term government work, to fortify the country's reputation and its soft power. Importantly (despite these challenges), since it can call on both an energy-based economy and diversification efforts, the UAE's economy is remaining resilient. As for Qatar, despite its initiatives for diversifying the economy, as demonstrated, it continues to rely heavily on its energy resources. For this reason, the 'globalised' threat of COVID-19 had less impact on the former state. Considering such impacts on states' economies, the strategy of diversifying the economy may be reviewed by states' policymakers.

Qatar and, particularly, the UAE, have effectively used their capacities, strong economy and relatively low incidences of COVID-19, to provide humanitarian aid globally. The COVID-19 pandemic has helped the UAE in particular to emerging as a potential 'strong' state globally, as it tackled the pandemic in alliance with other states globally. The pandemic has also demonstrated that military alliances in such times are arguably ineffective, not unchangeable and in some ways less significant. Overall, in such times, countries can increase their influence by working in collaboration with other states to tackle a specific threat and to demonstrate humanitarian policies. Moreover, at the policy-maker level, the pandemic illustrates how the UAE leadership further developed policies on foreign aid, offering help broadly globally. Meanwhile, Qatar seems to have mainly offered help to its friendly states and political allies. The state also continued to rely on governmental and non-governmental spread of foreign aid, relying on Ministries and charitable organisations, and state-owned Qatar Airways, institutions which have been often reliable for conducting Qatar's foreign policies. Therefore, as both cases illustrate, such uncertain times offer opportunities for states, and they can diversify and develop new policies and wider reach (as the UAE case study illustrates) or rely on 'trusted' policies (as the Qatar case study suggests).

Limitations and Directions for Future Research

Due to space limitation, this chapter does not discuss the so-called Great Powers response to COVID-19 on the basis of neo-realist theory. However, these states have been particularly hard hit by COVID-19. For example, Russia meets almost all the key indicators for neo-realist measures of power in being equipped to deal with threats, traditionally conceived. The COVID-19 pandemic, however, demonstrates that some of these same capacities can be disadvantages, where large territories and populations generate problematic complexity. Russia is my example here because MENA states cannot be fully characterised as Great Powers; additionally Russia, with its Muslim population of more than 20m, can be seen as useful for further comparative analyses.

Despite good early measures taken when the spread of the pandemic started, Russia faced an extended period of lockdown. The number of cases started to increase rapidly. To illustrate, on 8 May, the country had the seventh-highest number of people infected with COVID-19, and only in a few days, on 11 May, it was the fifth highest. The number of cases has been steadily growing, bringing Russia to third position of number cases globally by the beginning of summer. That might be explained by lack of action in March. However, it seems that the massive number of COVID-19 cases is also related to its key characteristics as a state, including its vast population and the world's largest territory.

Within the Russian Federation, the most affected areas were also the most populated places. The top three were regions with the highest population, as higher population means a more concentrated and mobile population, which increases the rate of infection. Unsurprisingly, the first was Moscow (total population 12,537,954, with 175,829 coronavirus cases recorded), second was Moscow Oblast (total population 759,9647 with 37,503 cases) and third Saint Petersburg (5,467,808 and 15,215, respectively). The death statistics also confirm this trend to an extent – the first is Moscow (2,330) and the second is Moscow Oblast (400). The exception is that the Dagestan Republic comes in third (Statista, 2020). The Republic of Dagestan has a population of only 2,910,249, mostly Muslim. The reasons for this discrepancy are related to another 'disadvantage' of neo-realist power indicators, as will be detailed below. Russia's vast territory is not only difficult to control in circumstances such as COVID-19 where coordinated action is required but also incorporates regions with very different regions, in an essentially multinational state.

Russia's territory, which is divided into 85 federal subjects, is subject to the variations of limitations of some regions, especially in regard to health systems and more poorly trained medical personnel. Medical unpreparedness to treat COVID-19 is illustrated in the case of Bashkortostan, half of the population of which is Muslims. In April, Bashkortostan had recorded 1 infected person, but this spread to 170 people within a few days. Among the infected were doctors, who had to stay at a hospital in quarantine because they were still obliged to treat patients (1tv.ru, 2020). Moreover, the different training experience of doctors in different regions might be demonstrated by news reports from June 10. On behalf of the mayor of Moscow, six Moscow medical teams, which are more advanced in training expertise, were deployed to support doctors in North Ossetia-Alania, Ingushetia, Trans-Baikal Territory, Dagestan, Vladimir and Pskov. In total, about 40 paramedics from the leading hospitals of the capital are expected to arrive to replace doctors in these regions (RBC.ru, 2020).

Moreover, the quick spread of the pandemic put more pressure on the regional governance, because the federal government has not yet become capable of controlling the enormous size of Russia centrally. Partly, the complexity of such a task rests on ethnic diversity. Not only ethnic Russians but more than 185 different ethnicities are represented in the country. The role of traditions and social structure in a multinational Russia has affected the ability to control the spread of the pandemic, as in the case of the Muslim Republic of Dagestan. The rates of mortality and infection have been high in the republic, as noted earlier, which is mainly explained by its social structure and traditions. A significant part of the inhabitants go to work from villages to the cities of Dagestan and to other regions and then return. By tradition, after returning, people need to meet with relatives, neighbours and friends and this always involves dozens of handshakes. The situation was complicated by the tradition of very large weddings, funerals and birth celebrations, which can generate significant and prolonged crowds. There is some evidence that funerals contributed to the infection rate in many ways: after *taziyats* (condolences procedures), massive outbreaks of infection were recorded (Kazenin and Starodubrovskaya, 2020).

While neo-realists' measurements of power, especially based on the size and number of population, proved to be disadvantages for Russia during COVID-19, an alternative view of neo-realist literature, touching on possible ways for increasing influence during the pandemic has been suggested above. Providing foreign aid has become an additional indicator of power. Russia provided foreign aid to Italy, including protective equipment and ventilators labelled 'From Russia with love' and 122 Russian army doctors. Russia provided medical aid to Belarus, Serbia, Armenia and Ecuador (Tchoubar, 2020). The country also sent a plane, full of medical supplies, including masks and medical equipment, to the US (Roth, 2020). Such 'strategic' initiatives are connected by observers with Russia's 'attempt to inherit [the] geopolitical role of the USSR' (Loshak, 2020).

Therefore, examination of so-called Great Powers can be important for further development of the argument, that the neo-realist tradition does not adequately illustrate the patterns and possibilities of world politics: 'smallness' can rather serve as an advantage during such pandemics (and possible other periods of uncertainty). Moreover, it is important to acknowledge the specific responses of particular emirates or regions and federal governance to fight COVID-19, based on the specific characteristics of places. For example, Dagestan's traditions affected the ability of central Russian control to reduce the spread of the virus, with social interactions being a primary route of transmission. That the study of the small GCC states given above (with similar traditions) did not indicate the same degree of spread over the longer term shows the importance of understanding local conditions and responding accordingly. Finally, Russia's illustration of foreign aid during the pandemic, which was still less than that given by the discussed so-called 'small states', so further research can further demonstrate that differentiation of states on the basis of 'weak' and 'strong' is no longer adequate within world politics.

Conclusions

The neo-realist approach to International Relations theory considers small states as inherently 'weak', based on a quantitative view of capacity and power. However, an examination of small GCC states challenges this perception, especially where their wealth and resources can be translated into better internal controls and consolidated alliances to tackle this pandemic (by offering foreign aid). As illustrated, the Arab Spring allowed the policymakers of the GCC states to emerge as regional players and increase the GCC states' power and influence. Almost ten years afterwards, another unprecedented global event, the pandemic offered them an opportunity to spread this influence globally. In contrast to the neo-realist view, the GCC states, as demonstrated in the case studies of the UAE and Qatar, tackled the pandemic more effectively and have reported lower numbers of infections and consequently deaths. At the same time, wealth served as a vital power tool for offering foreign aid to both 'strong' and 'weak' states. In other words, such unprecedented events can provide an opportunity for policymakers to implement active foreign policies and even power projections. Overall, the pandemic, through the lens of foreign aid, has underlined the emergence of the UAE, particularly, and to a lesser extent, Qatar, on the global stage as potentially 'strong' states. Therefore, this chapter demonstrates how the political status of the small GCC states has transformed globally, due to state characteristics and the actions implemented by their policymakers.

References

1tv.ru (2020) 'V bashkirii rassledyut' obstoyatelstva masovogo zaracheniya v krupneishei bol'nice respubliki'. https://www.1tv.ru/news/2020-04-11/383710-v_bashkirii_rassleduyut_obstoyatelstva_massovogo_zarazheniya_v_krupneyshey_bolnitse_respubliki

Aburumman, A. (2020) *COVID-19 Impact and Survival Strategy in Business Tourism Market: The Example of the UAE MICE Industry.* https://www.nature.com/articles/s41599-020-00630-8

Al-Arabiya (2021) *Coronavirus: Russian COVID-19 Vaccine Trials Begin in Abu Dhabi.* https://english.alarabiya.net/en/coronavirus/2021/01/07/Coronavirus-Russian-COVID-19-vaccine-trials-begin-in-Abu-Dhabi

Al-Jazeera (2020a) *Record Infections, Few Deaths: How Qatar Has Tackled COVID-19.* https://www.aljazeera.com/news/2020/8/26/record-infections-few-deaths-how-qatar-has-tackled-covid-19

Al Mezaini, K. (2012) *The UAE and Foreign Policy: Foreign Aid, Identities, and Interests.* London: Routledge.

Alshamsi, R. (2020) *A Blessing in Disguise: UAE's Possible Scenarios for a Post-COVID-19 World.* https://www.e-ir.info/2020/08/19/a-blessing-in-disguise-uaes-possible-scenarios-for-a-post-covid-19-world/

Amer, A. (2019) *Qatar Pledges to Keep Money Pipeline Open to Gaza Strip.* https://www.al-monitor.com/pulse/originals/2019/02/palestine-israel-gaza-hamas-qatar-grant-billion-amount-aid.html

Blas, J. and Arkhipov, I. (2020) *Russia and Saudi Arabia Step Up Oil Diplomacy.* https://www.bloomberg.com/news/articles/2020-10-17/russia-saudi-arabia-ready-to-keep-energy-market-stable-kremlin

Braw, E. (2020) Europe's Coronavirus Response: Selfish Member States and Active Institutions, *RUSI.* https://rusi.org/commentary/europe-coronavirus-response-selfish-member-states-and-active-institutions (Accessed: 17 June 2020).

CGTN (2020) *China Says It Has Help Over 130 Countries and Intl Organizations Fight Covid-19 Pandemic.* https://news.cgtn.com/news/2020-04-10/Chinese-experts-share-experiences-in-combating-COVID-19-PzeGMp0uHe/index.html

Clarke, C. and Payne, A. (1987) *Politics, Security and Development in Small States.* Allen & Unwin, London.

Conn, D. (2017) *Michael Garcia's Fifa Report Eases Russia and Qatar Wold Cup Fear.* https://www.theguardian.com/football/2017/jun/27/fifa-secret-report-world-cup-2022-leaked

Dillon, J. (2018) *Bayern Munich Deepen Their Ties to Qatar.* https://www.bavarian-footballworks.com/2018/2/22/17038682/bayern-munich-qatar-airways-lufthansa-hamad-airport-sponsor-champions-league-finances-revenue

Elman, M. (1995) The Foreign Policies of Small States: Challenging Neorealism in Its Own Backyard, *British Journal of Political Science,* 25 (2), 171–217.

Fattah, Z. (2020) Dubai to Ease Movement Curbs as Malls: Offices Slowly Reopen', *Bloomberg.* https://www.bloomberg.com/news/articles/2020-04-23/dubai-to-ease-movement-curbs-as-malls-offices-slowly-reopen

Fromherz, A. (2012) *Qatar: A Modern History.* London: Tauris.

Galeeva, D. (2020) Balancing Adversaries: Russian Policy in the Gulf and the Role of Russian Muslims, *LSE blog.* https://blogs.lse.ac.uk/mec/2020/01/02/balancing-adversaries-russian-policy-in-the-gulf-and-the-role-of-russian-muslims/

Garcia, B. and Amara, M. (2013) Media Perceptions of Arab Investment in European Football Clubs: The Case of Malaga and Paris Saint-Germain, *Sport and EU Review,* 5 (1), 5–20.

GardaWorld, (2020) *UAE: Travel Restrictions Eased for Residents of Abu Dhabi July 4/Update 49.* https://www.garda.com/crisis24/news-alerts/358091/uae-travel-restrictions-eased-for-residents-of-abu-dhabi-july-4-update-49

GHD (2020) *Qatar Field Hospital Designed from Scratch in Less than Two Weeks.* https://www.ghd.com/en/news/qatar-field-hospital-designed-from-scratch-in-less-than-two-weeks.aspx

Gössling, S., Scott, D., and Hall, C. (2020) Pandemics, Tourism and Global Change: A Rapid Assessment of COVID-19. *Sustain Tourism.* 29 (1), 1–20. https://doi.org/10.1080/09669582.2020.1758708

Government of Dubai Media Office (2020) *Supreme Committee of Crisis and Disaster Management Announces New Air Travel Protocols.* https://mediaoffice.ae/en/news/2020/June/21-06/Supreme-Committee-of-Crisis-and-Disaster-Management-announces-new-air-travel-protocols

Gray, M. (2011) *A Theory of "Late Rentierism" in the Arab States of the Gulf.* https://repository.library.georgetown.edu/bitstream/handle/10822/558291/CIRSOccasionalPaper7MatthewGray2011.pdf

Haza, R. (2020) Public Beaches and Malls in Ras Al Khaimah to Reopen from Thursday, *The National.* https://www.thenational.ae/uae/public-beaches-and-malls-in-ras-al-khaimah-to-reopen-from-thursday-1.1025765

Hoffman, A. (2020) Is Securitization the Solution to Containing the Coronavirus Crisis? *IR in the Age of Coronavirus.* https://irintheageofcorona.com/is-securitization-the-solution-to-containing-the-coronavirus-crisis/

IMF (2020) *World Economic Outlook a Long and Difficult Ascent.* https://www.imf.org/en/Publications/WEO/Issues/2020/09/30/world-economic-outlook-october-2020

International Cooperation Department Ministry of Foreign Affairs. (2020) *The State of Qatar's Aid to Friendly Countries to Confront the Emerging Corona Virus 'Covid-19'.* https://www.ohchr.org/Documents/Events/GoodPracticesCoronavirus/qatar-submission-covid19.pdf

Ismail, N. W. (2020). Digital trade facilitation and bilateral trade in selected Asian countries. *Studies in Economics and Finance* (ahead-of-print). https://doi.org/10.1108/sef-10-2019-0406

Jones, M. (2020) *Covid-19 in Qatar: Well Versed in Crisis Management.* https://www.qu.edu.qa/static-file/qu/research/Gulf%20Studies/documents/Gulf%20Insights%2021.pdf

Kamrava, M. (ed.) (2016) *Fragile Politics Weak States in the Greater Middle East.* New York: Oxford University Press.

Kazenin, K. and Starodubrovskaya, I. (2020) Simptomy Nedoverya: Pochemu Dagestan Tyachelo Perechivaet Epidemiu', *RBC.ru.* https://www.rbc.ru/opinions/politics/21/05/2020/5ec559ce9a79474af0cf7019

Keohane, R. (1969). Lilliputians Dilemmas: Small States in International Politics. *International Organization*, 23 (2), 291–310.

Khaleej Times (2021) *Covid-19 Vaccine in UAE: 80,683 People Vaccinated Last 24 Hours.* https://www.khaleejtimes.com/coronavirus-pandemic/covid-19-vaccine-in-uae-80683-people-vaccinated-in-last-24-hours

Loshak, V. (2020) Posle Virusa Peremeny Neizbechny, No Gotova Li K Nim Vlast'? *Ogonek, 19*, 5614, May 2020, 8.

Masaryk, T. (1966) *The Problem of Small Nations in the European Crisis.* London: University of London, School of Slavonic and East European Studies.

Naar, I. (2020a) Dubai Eases Coronavirus Restrictions as it Marks Ramadan: 10 Questions Answered', *Al-Arabiya Englis.* https://english.alarabiya.net/en/coronavirus/2020/04/24/Dubai-eases-coronavirus-restrictions-as-it-marks-Ramadan-10-questions-answered

Naar, I. (2020b) Coronavirus: Dubai Launches 'Dubai Assured' Stamp for Tourism, Retail Establishments, *Al-Arabiya English.* https://english.alarabiya.net/en/coronavirus/2020/07/19/Coronavirus-Dubai-launches-Dubai-assured-stamp-for-tourism-retail-establishments.html

RBC.ru (2020) Glav vrach Bol'nichy V Kommunarke Otravitsya Na Pomosh' Medikam Dagestana. https://amp.rbc.ru/rbcnews/society/10/06/2020/5ee0a5969a794796db-b29675?utm_source=tw_rbc&__twitter_impression=true

Reliefweb (2020) Covid-19 Pandemic: Government Strengthens Humanitarian Efforts. https://reliefweb.int/report/world/covid-19-pandemic-government-strengthens-humanitarian-efforts

Reynolds, D. (2020) *Hundreds of Millions in U.S. Foreign Aid to Combat COVID-19.* https://uk.usembassy.gov/hundreds-of-millions-in-u-s-foreign-aid-to-combat-covid-19/

Roma, A.S. (2018) *Roma Announce Qatar Airways as Main Global Partner.* https://www.asroma.com/en/news/2018/4/roma-announce-qatar-airways-as-main-global-partner

Roth, A. (2020) Coronavirus: Russia Sends Plane Full of Medical Supplies to US, *The Guardian.* https://www.theguardian.com/world/2020/apr/01/coronavirus-russia-sends-plane-full-of-medical-supplies-to-us

Rudoren, J. (2012) *Qatar's Visits Gaza, Pledging $ 400 Million to Hamas.* https://www.nytimes.com/2012/10/24/world/middleeast/pledging-400-million-qatari-emir-makes-historic-visit-to-gaza-strip.html?mtrref=www.google.com&gwh=A0FCBB620858827DD1FA5227735F1C8A&gwt=pay

Ryan, P. (2020) Coronavirus: Joggers, Dog Walkers and Cyclists Return to Abu Dhabi Corniche, *The National.* https://www.thenational.ae/uae/coronavirus-joggers-dog-walkers-and-cyclists-return-to-abu-dhabi-corniche-1.1033331

Shirka, H. (2020) Abu Dhabi Hotels to Reopen Beaches, *The National.* https://www.thenational.ae/lifestyle/travel/abu-dhabi-hotels-to-reopen-beaches-1.1027239

Statista (2020) *COVID-19 Deaths Worldwide as of June 17, 2020, by Country.* https://www.statista.com/statistics/1093256/novel-coronavirus-2019ncov-deaths-worldwide-by-country/

Tchoubar, P. (2020) Covid-19: A Test for Russia's African Ambitions', *European Council on Foreign Relations.* https://www.ecfr.eu/article/commentary-covid-19-a-test-for-russias-african-ambitions

The Guardian (2019) *Qatar to Send $480m to Help Palestinians in West Bank and Gaza.* https://www.theguardian.com/world/2019/may/07/qatar-send-480m-help-palestinians-west-bank-gaza-israel-ceasefire (Accessed: 20 January 2020).

The Jerusalem Post (2019) *Qatar to Send Delayed $ 15 Million Payment to Gaza.* https://www.jpost.com/Arab-Israeli-Conflict/Qatar-to-send-delayed-15-million-payment-to-Gaza-578060

The Peninsula (2020) *Qatar Designated 5 Hospitals, 4 Testing Centers and an Isolation Hospital for Covid-19 Cases: Public Health Director.* https://thepeninsulaqatar.com/article/28/04/2020/Qatar-designated-5-hospitals,-4-testing-centers-and-an-isolation-hospital-for-Covid-19-cases-Public-Health-Director?__cf_chl_captcha_tk__ =1f4f9b1cfd807490d3988d9565a1abdce4c436b6–1609780511-0-Ad4rvA2lVXye 0bmZNNws3yeRXIDLcR0OSEUukgK7K4LeyQab5SzKBZenPGAlem6qs-CNgi3t9RSCxY_TMbTUzqn5eQlJiABTLxJ1nX1c4wrYGLvRtv5EA8CsTBzyk68a-BwNW2uaPl9ISCOkXUAc1p7btj5gq-0nQW8674BBrUAylQ6kfVDR3wnYSp5qe-o35zQP1HwBvw_WBbTQ0gFcEd7Rbo1LTfxGtmvlrSOuxnTXwQtCf4_-5nBg-PevDGGWo5ias3N_jpuH_LMBEiCibVbIXp96L2frgEn9hB-UIaluTKbKB-sC5-ynNhyLwVcE_YJeMojfTm1h7hEEX6971_m0uQ4ZyP3mQW8RazmzT-GyEQqy3xG94qmlleLcuwl94xdDGuSUrbplJxd8ILMheZlo4BNyxOf5FT8gjVne-CYCGvqdSqN2GANcx8C-r82ruroLpC-PnHfzz21uUDlnxYp8wzNIfKi7CPb-jBA03fsWwcF62jLSJ76hfVW1LqaWF6HDlNmh-0zA0t2u3mZJRr2AhIZEXas-yCuzVZ9CCUijaY93sKl3pGXYH3Mnx3m4JckaGbUVGeeGXeqj99hvvfBJKs-G44YRUCXQyS0rm1mTthpwEbf1eE2pbsJ_wynNUkcAskbqbhhYjdgUiEB-m908H8NjZtSd7MGl2LCv6jIYX8tnsfRkaB4d21PTAiEyuBKN96Wl2MH8A

Trading Economics (2019) *Qatar GDP.* https://tradingeconomics.com/qatar/gdp

Ulrichsen, C. (2014) *Qatar and the Arab Spring.* London: Hurst & Company.

Vital, D. (1967) *The Inequality of States: A Study of the Small Power in International Relations.* Oxford: Clarendon P.

Waltz, K.N. (1979). *Theory of International Politics.* Reading, MA: Addison-Wesley.

Watanabe, L. (2017) Gulf States' Engagement in North Africa: The Role of Foreign Aid, in: Almezaini, S. and Rickli, J.-M. (eds.) *The Small Gulf States Foreign and Security Policies Before and After the Arab Spring.* New York: Routledge, 168–181.

Worldometers (2020a) *United Arab Emirates.* https://www.worldometers.info/coronavirus/country/united-arab-emirates/

Worldometers (2020b) *Qatar.* https://www.worldometers.info/coronavirus/country/qatar/

Wright, S. (2016) The Emergence of Qatar as a Small State Actor. *Critique Internationale, 2* (71), 73–88.

Young, K. (2019) What's Yours Is Mine: Gulf SWFs as Barometer of State-Society Relations. The Politics of Rentier States in the Gulf, *POMEPS Studies, 33*, 44–50.

4   Jordan and Tunisia Lose Their Luster

An Institutional and Policy Journey against COVID-19

Nejla Ben Mimoune

Introduction

As the coronavirus pandemic hit the globe, countries have implemented different policy and institutional measures in an attempt to control the outbreak. Jordan and Tunisia's initial responses to COVID-19 were considered among the most effective in the Middle East and North Africa (MENA) region, even though the two countries had healthcare systems that were less well-developed and financed compared to Gulf countries. Shortly after the first COVID-19 cases were confirmed, both countries moved swiftly to implement a number of comprehensive measures including border closure, the suspension of in-person classes, night curfews, and nationwide lockdowns.[1] For instance, Jordan's pandemic lockdown was considered among the strictest worldwide.[2] As a result, by early May 2020, Jordan and Tunisia had initially succeeded in containing the outbreak and flattening the first curve – a milestone that was reached before other neighboring countries. However, while managing to successfully contain the outbreak, the national lockdowns had serious economic repercussions in both countries, which had previously already been suffering from several structural economic problems. Under these pressures, the two governments started lifting restrictions, resuming economic activities, and opening their borders. These actions, in turn, led initially to a gradual increase in the daily numbers of new COVID-19 cases and deaths. By the fall of 2020, the numbers increased significantly, indicating much larger new waves in both countries. To mitigate the second and third waves of the outbreak, Jordan and Tunisia launched COVID-19 inoculation programs during the first quarter of 2021. To date, around 17% of Jordan's population and less than 7% of Tunisia's have received at least one dose of COVID-19 vaccine.[3]

Jordan and Tunisia continue to struggle to find the right balance between measures halting the outbreak and limiting its economic repercussions. With the coronavirus lasting for the long haul, what are the next response measures in Jordan and Tunisia? How will they strike the balance between the epidemiological and economic situations? This chapter looks at Jordan and Tunisia's journeys responding to the coronavirus pandemic. It examines

DOI: 10.4324/9781003266259-4

the different institutional and policy measures taken to control the virus and inspects attempts at limiting its economic repercussions.

Is Too Early to Celebrate?

By the end of February 2020, several MENA countries had confirmed their first cases of COVID-19. At the time and as a precaution, Jordan had started implementing airport screenings and imposing hotel quarantines for incoming travelers. Yet shortly after March 2, the kingdom reported its first confirmed coronavirus infection. As the cases gradually increased afterwards, the government started imposing increasingly serious measures to limit the outbreak. For instance, it announced a state of emergency and activated the National Defense Law 13 of 1992, granting the prime minister wider powers to enact needed measures to control the pandemic. All international flights from and to Queen Alia International Airport were suspended between March 17 and September 8, 2020, with the exception of few repatriation flights. Once international flights had resumed, passengers had to adhere to special travel measures such as presenting a negative Polymerase Chain Reaction (PCR) test within 72 hours of travel. Meanwhile, land borders remained mostly open for commercial trade only. The academic year for 2019–2020 was ended in mid-March, when classes were initially suspended and then later canceled for the remainder of the school year. In addition, Jordan implemented strict physical distancing measures and limited movement within the kingdom. It had imposed night curfews and one of the strictest national lockdowns, with the military ensuring people adhered to these procedures. All economic activity, cultural events, and group religious practices stopped until mid-April, when restrictions started being lifted gradually. By early May 2020, Jordan had lifted most restrictions following the flattening of the first curve of COVID-19.[4] At the time, only 461 total COVID-19 case (45.63 per million population) and nine cumulative deaths had been confirmed,[5] an incidence much lower than the more capable Gulf countries.[6] To communicate COVID-19 statistics and new measures, the minister of health, minister of state for media affairs, and the director of the Coronavirus Crisis Cell addressed the public in regular news conferences from the office of the prime minister. These briefings have been also published on the Ministry of Health's COVID-19 dedicated website along with the social media pages of the ministry and Cabinet.[7]

Jordan's initial swift response had been classified among the strictest in the world.[8] The strictness of a government's response to the coronavirus pandemic over time can be captured by the Stringency Index of the Oxford COVID-19 Government Response Tracker. This composite index is based on nine different measure indicators capturing border closure, school suspension, and business shutdown, among others. It ranges on a scale of zero to 100, with 100 being the strictest response.[9] Shortly after the COVID-19 outbreak hit Jordan, it had reached the top score in terms of response strictness on this index, and when compared to other MENA countries, such swift and rigorous intervention kept Jordan's initial COVID-19 infection rates at bay.[10]

Jordan had benefited from the pre-existing National Committee for Epidemics, which was established in 1984 to research epidemics in the world. It included healthcare professionals and government officials and consulted with various entities such as the Ministry of Health, research establishments, and the World Health Organization (WHO). The body spearheaded the kingdom's COVID-19 response, convening regularly to assess the ongoing epidemiological situation and recommending policy action accordingly. In addition, Jordan had created a specialized Coronavirus Crisis Cell within its National Center for Security and Crisis Management (NCSCM). The latter is an umbrella organization established in 2015 under the Royal Court to coordinate the actions of national institutions during national crises. Furthermore, the Cabinet had created inter-ministerial teams to advise on the various aspects of the crisis, including health care, border control, social protection, and education and work continuity. The military also played an important role in coordinating response efforts, implementing the directions of the prime minister under the Defense Law and making sure people adhered to lockdown and curfew measures.[11]

In addition, Jordan's relatively capable health sector had initially played a major role in limiting COVID-19 deaths and the case fatality rate (CFR)[12]. In 2018, health expenditure amounted to 8.8% of Jordan's gross domestic product (GDP).[13] Compared to Egypt and Morocco, the Hashemite Kingdom had higher current health expenditure per capita, although lower than neighboring Lebanon or Tunisia.[14] Furthermore, to harness the country's full potential, Jordan's top leaders called for collaborations among all stakeholders, including the Ghiath and Nadia Sukhitan Foundation, the TechWorks Initiative of the Crown Prince Foundation, as well as the private health sector. For instance, thanks to a well-managed collaboration with private sector laboratories, the kingdom succeeded in scaling up its testing capacities significantly.[15]

Tunisia was another MENA best performer during the initial wave of the coronavirus pandemic. On March 2, 2020, the country had recorded its first confirmed COVID-19 case. At the time, the republic had been already in a national state of emergence since a terrorist attack took place in 2015. By mid-March, the government had started acting swiftly to limit the spread of infections. The parliament designated the prime minister to spearhead the country's response to COVID-19. Like Jordan, classes were initially suspended and later mostly canceled throughout the 2019–2020 school year.

The exception was for high school seniors and university students who resumed classes for few weeks by the end of May before taking baccalaureate and final exams, respectively. Tunisia had also closed all borders from

March 16 until June 27, 2020, apart from few repatriation flights for Tunisians returning from overseas. Once the borders opened again, the government imposed special COVID-19 travel measures on incoming passengers depending on the epidemiological situation in their countries of residence. Countries were classified into three categories: green, orange, and red, with the first group not subject to any COVID-19 precautionary measures. Like Jordan, Tunisia also imposed nightly curfews and a national lockdown to limit people's movement and social gatherings, thereby slowing the domestic spread of the virus. All cultural events, non-essential economic activities, and group prayers were suspended until early May, when a gradual deconfinement strategy was initiated. All activities had resumed to a 100% capacity by mid-June.[16] At the start of the deconfinement, Tunisia had confirmed 1,018 cumulative COVID-19 cases (87.05 per million population, nearly double that of Jordan) and 43 total deaths,[17] an incidence higher at the time than Jordan, Iraq, and Egypt, yet lower than neighboring Morocco or the five Gulf countries.[18] Representatives of the Ministry of Health together with a crisis communication team held regular press conferences broadcasted through national television and radio channels to update the public about the epidemiological situation of the country and communicate new measures. These updates were also published through a COVID-19 specific website and the Facebook pages of the Ministry of Health and the Republic Presidency.[19]

On March 25, 2020, the Tunisian government created the National Coronavirus Response Authority (NCRA) to centralize and unify preventive and control measures. The body led the country's COVID-19 action plan and coordinated the response measures within the country's 24 governorates. The NCRA was supervised by the prime minister and included representatives of the different government branches such as the ministers of health, interior, social affairs, and transportation and technologies, among others. Furthermore, and like Jordan, Tunisia had benefited from its pre-existing institutions. For instance, the National Observatory of New and Emerging Diseases, which was founded in 2005 under the Ministry of Health, provided research input and guidance on how to respond to the outbreak. In addition, the Permanent National Committee for Disaster Prevention, Response, and Relief Organization, established in 1993 under the supervision of the Ministry of Interior, worked with the NCRA to coordinate and unify response measures. The police and military forces had also played an important role in ensuring enforcement.[20]

The strictness of Tunisia's response to the pandemic is captured by the Oxford COVID-19 Government Response Tracker's Stringency Index. Although the index did not reach the top score like Jordan, Tunisia's swift initial response succeeded in keeping infection rates low throughout the end of August 2020 (see Figures 4.1 and 4.2), which at the time was significantly lower than other MENA countries.[21]

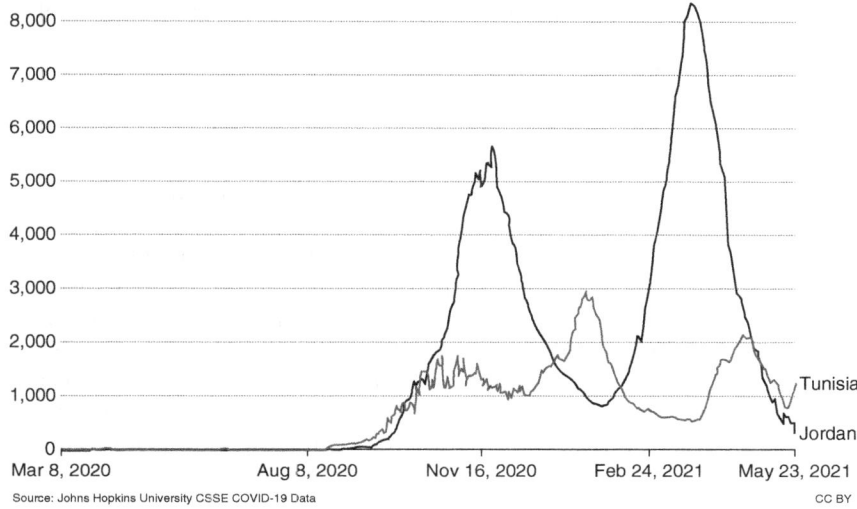

Figure 4.1 Daily new confirmed COVID-19 cases: Jordan and Tunisia

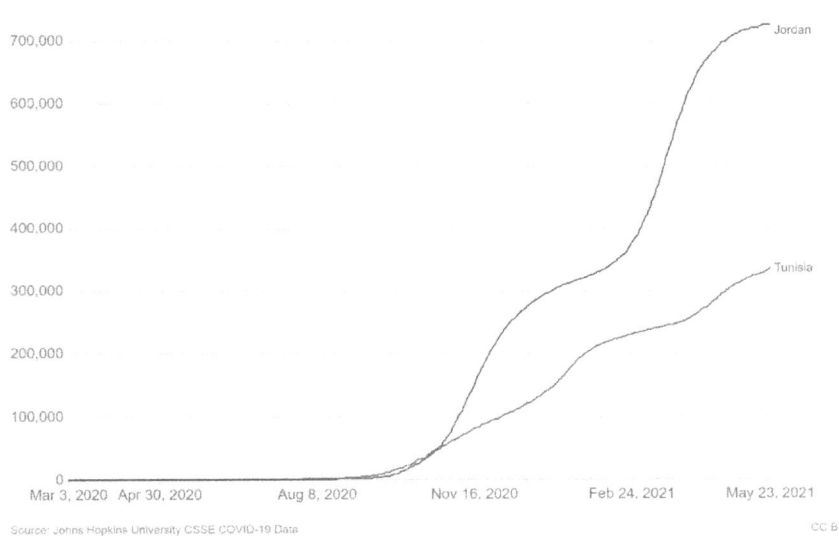

Figure 4.2 Cumulative confirmed COVID-19 cases: Jordan and Tunisia

Tunisia had a relatively strong public health infrastructure, with several university and regional hospitals, along with more than 100 district hospitals dispersed across the country.[22] The public healthcare system was capable to handle the outbreak in its first phase, when the number of cases was limited, and it managed to keep COVID-19 deaths and case fatality rate initially at bay (see Figures 4.3–4.5).

In 2018, current health expenditure was 7.3% of Tunisia's GDP.[23] Although, as a percentage of GDP, Tunisia's health expenditure was less than Jordan's, in dollar terms it was higher than the latter's, yet still lower than Lebanon's.[24] To reinforce its capacities, the government had also called on the private sector and civil society to collaborate and support the health sector. They both contributed to the production of medical supplies and personal protective equipment (PPE). In addition, private sector laboratories supported the very limited public capacities in terms of COVID-19 screening. Yet, Tunisia's testing capacities remained very limited compared to other countries of the region, including Jordan (see Figures 4.6 and 4.7).[25]

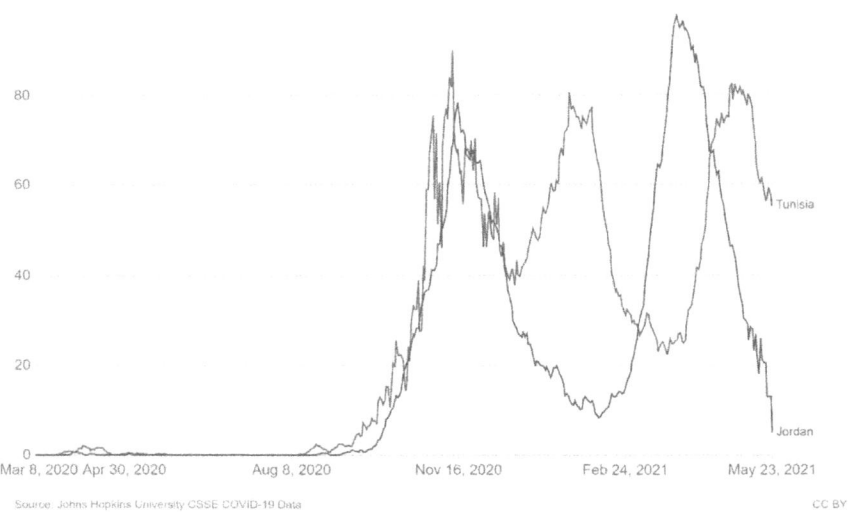

Source: Johns Hopkins University CSSE COVID-19 Data   CC BY

Figure 4.3 Daily new confirmed COVID-19 deaths: Jordan and Tunisia

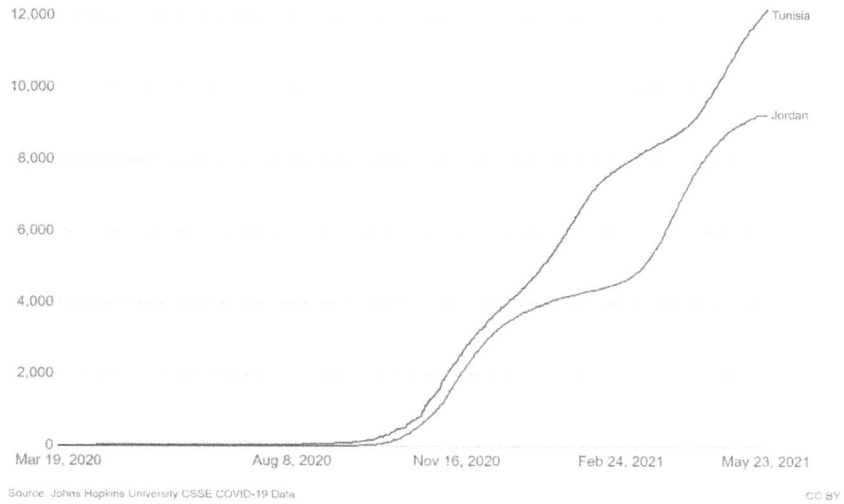

Figure 4.4 Cumulative confirmed COVID-19 deaths: Jordan and Tunisia

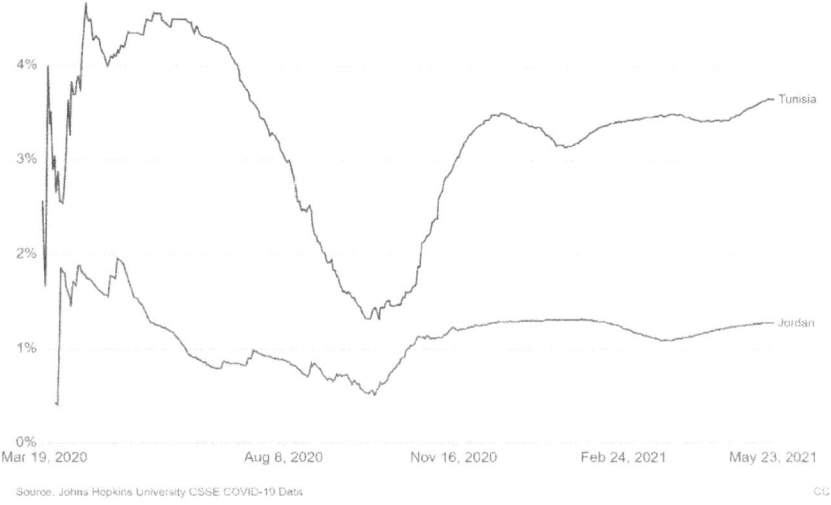

Figure 4.5 Case fatality rate of the ongoing COVID-19 pandemic: Jordan and Tunisia

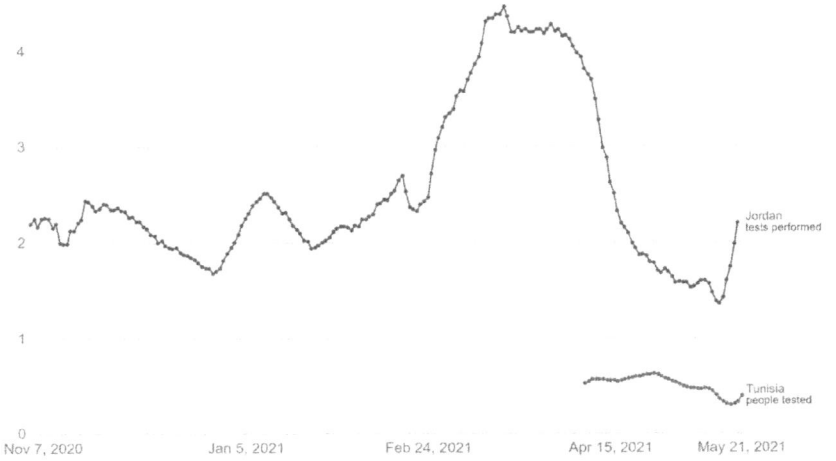

Source: Official data collated by Our World in Data – Last updated 21 May, 15:00 (London time)
Note: Comparisons of testing data across countries are affected by differences in the way the data are reported. Daily data is interpolated for countries not reporting testing data on a daily basis. Details can be found at our Testing Dataset page.

OurWorldInData.org/coronavirus • CC BY

Figure 4.6 Daily COVID-19 tests per thousand people: Jordan and Tunisia

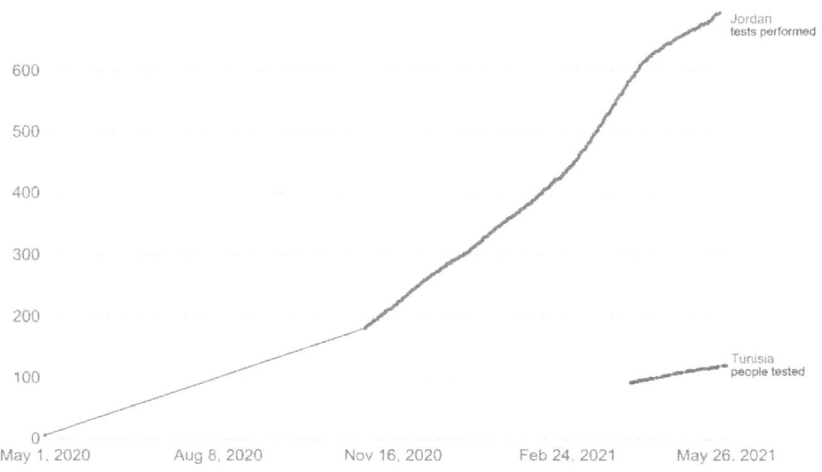

Source: Official sources collated by Our World in Data
Note: Comparisons of testing data across countries are affected by differences in the way the data are reported. Details can be found at our Testing Dataset page.

OurWorldInData.org/coronavirus • CC BY

Figure 4.7 Total COVID-19 tests per 1,000 people: Jordan and Tunisia

It Is Not All Glamorous After All

Economic Repercussions

The COVID-19 pandemic together with the imposed lockdowns and restrictions has shaken the global economy. Most business activities went through prolonged shutdown periods, affecting production levels, employment, and incomes. Already suffering from several structural economic challenges, Jordan and Tunisia were no different from the other economies. For instance, the Hashemite Kingdom has a unique demographic structure with refugees representing about one-third of the population and many of whom are unregistered. This exerts additional pressure on the limited available resources, especially with a significant loss in remittances due to the returning Jordanian workers from the Gulf countries amid the pandemic. Additionally, Jordan suffers from a crippling budget deficit and public debt that are on the rise.[26] Tunisia, on the other hand, suffers from heavy reliance on the tourism sector, which represented 14.2% of 2019 GDP and directly employed around 11% of the workplace. Unfortunately, tourism is one of the most affected sectors globally by the coronavirus pandemic.[27] In Tunisia, the sector's revenues dropped by 65% in 2020 compared to the 2019 levels.[28] The country was also suffering from a large budget deficit and high levels of external debts, driven by low revenues and a high civil service salary bill.[29]

Following the pandemic, the economic situation in both countries worsened. Jordan reported a 2% economic contraction for 2020, while Tunisia's economy contracted by 8.8%, the largest downturn since Tunisia's independence, yet lower than the economic contraction in Oman, Iraq, Lebanon, and Palestine.[30] In 2021, real GDP growth is predicted to bounce back to 2% and 3.8% for Jordan and Tunisia, respectively. The 2020 fiscal deficit was estimated at 11.5% of GDP in Tunisia following a lower tax intake and a higher service salary bill driven by additional hiring in the health sector. Additionally, general government debt levels as a percentage of GDP increased to 88.5% and 87.6% in Jordan and Tunisia, respectively, and are estimated to further rise in 2021. Unemployment rates also increased compared to 2019 levels in both countries, disproportionally affecting informal sector workers, low-skilled laborers, women, and youth. In 2020, the overall unemployment increased by 3.6 points in Jordan reaching 22.7%,[31] and by 1.6 points in Tunisia marking 16.7%.[32] Poverty was also expected to increase because of the perceived economic slowdown. In Tunisia particularly, the increase in poverty was estimated to be between 7.3% and 11.9% in 2020.[33]

To mitigate some of these repercussions, both governments had announced several initiatives and support packages including reduction in key interest rate, extending loan and tax grace-payment plans, and establishing support funds for the most impacted businesses along with informal sector workers and vulnerable households.[34] Despite these important initiatives, the economic and social impact of the pandemic and lockdowns were large in both countries. Several scattered protests took place to object the situation, which were swiftly dispersed by the police. In Jordan particularly, teachers went on a nationwide strike following the government's decision to freeze civic service pay increases. In response, the police had arrested several members of the Jordanian Teachers Syndicate, which in return was met with further protests focusing on the economic situation, repression of syndicates, and government corruption.[35]

Crumbling Efforts

As Jordan and Tunisia eased up the strict restrictions of the first phase of the pandemic, COVID-19 cases started increasing gradually, then significantly escalating by the end of 2020. Several factors have contributed to this increase. First, both countries suffered from severe economic repercussions amid the first lockdown. Hence, as they eased the restrictions, they implemented much looser regulations post-confinement with the hope of picking up some of the lost economic gains. For instance, shortly after opening its borders, Tunisia did not impose any COVID-19 screening or confinement procedures on the incoming travelers of the green-list countries, which included most of Europe. In addition, both countries had laxer social gatherings and physical distancing regulations during the 2020 Eid al-Adha celebrations.[36] Another contributing factor was the 'pandemic fatigue' observed across the globe, which describes people's demotivation to follow the recommended protective practices such as wearing a mask, maintaining a hand hygiene, and retaining physical distance.[37]

Furthermore, while at the beginning of the pandemic both Jordanians and Tunisians showed high levels of trust in their governments and satisfaction with their abilities in controlling the outbreak, this decreased later with the social and economic impacts of the imposed restrictions, along with the surge in the number of COVID-19 cases and deaths. For instance, a poll conducted in June 2020 by the Strategic Studies Centre of the University of Jordan revealed that 92% of Jordanians considered the government's response to the pandemic as successful.[38] By October 2020, only 68% of Jordanians were satisfied with their government's response to the outbreak according to the fifth wave of the Arab Barometer.[39] Similarly in Tunisia, a national survey conducted in April 2020 revealed that 88% and 82% of Tunisians highly valued the response measures taken by the Ministry of Health and the security and military forces, respectively.[40] Meanwhile, when the fifth wave of the Arab Barometer was conducted in October, only 24% were satisfied with the government response.[41] With such lower trust and satisfaction levels, people are less likely to adhere to imposed measures.

As the outbreak continued past the deconfinement phase, COVID-19 cases and newer-more infectious strains spread across Jordan and Tunisia. In return, the exponentially rising infections had stretched the two countries' public healthcare systems beyond their capacities and limited their abilities of absorbing patients in need of intensive care. In return, the number of deaths increased significantly after the first phase. In Tunisia particularly, the healthcare system was drastically strained that the country had higher COVID-19 deaths than Jordan despite its lower total infections, hence rising its case fatality rate. Indeed, Tunisia has only around 500 intensive care beds across its 24 governorates. Meanwhile, more than 90 new patients needed hospitalization each day.[42] In addition, the public healthcare system suffers from severe geographic inequality in terms of resources distribution, including specialized doctors, intensive care units, updated medical equipment, and hospital access, favoring the Northern and coastal cities over the Southern and interior towns.[43] Jordan, on the other hand, suffered from an oxygen outage at the COVID-19 ward of one of its hospitals, which had led to the death of six patients, and the resignation of the health minister afterward.[44] With such proven limited capacities, people showed low satisfaction with the country healthcare system. Indeed, only 39% of Arab Barometer Tunisian respondents were satisfied with the system, compared to 63% of the Jordanians.[45]

The Road Ahead

Vaccination Drive

With the coronavirus most likely becoming an endemic virus, continuing to circulate in pockets globally, countries across the globe embarked on inoculation programs to limit its spread and lessen its symptoms. Jordan started its vaccination campaign on January 13, 2021, which was carried out by the Ministry of Health and the National Centre for Security and Crises Management. Jordan has established more than 70 vaccination centers across its land to accelerate the inoculation campaign, with more centers planned to be added. Any person living in Jordan, including refugees and asylum seekers, is eligible to receive the vaccine for free, provided they register on the health ministry's portal. Yet, priority is given to the elderly, individuals with underlying conditions, and health sector workers.[46] Currently, four different vaccines (Pfizer/BioNTech, Sputnik V, Oxford/AstraZeneca, and Beijing's Sinopharm) are approved for use in Jordan.[47] The kingdom had expected to receive more than 10 million doses of the vaccines in 2021, 2 million of which to be from the COVAX Facility.[48] The government had initially announced it intended to vaccinate more than 20% of the population, with 3 million doses of the vaccine to be administered by June 1, 2021.[49] However, by June 7, only 17.1% of the population had received at least one dose of the vaccine, corresponding to a total of 2.31 million administered shots (see Figures 4.8 and 4.9).[50]

Tunisia, on the other hand, started its national vaccination campaign much later than Jordan and the other MENA countries. On March 13, the

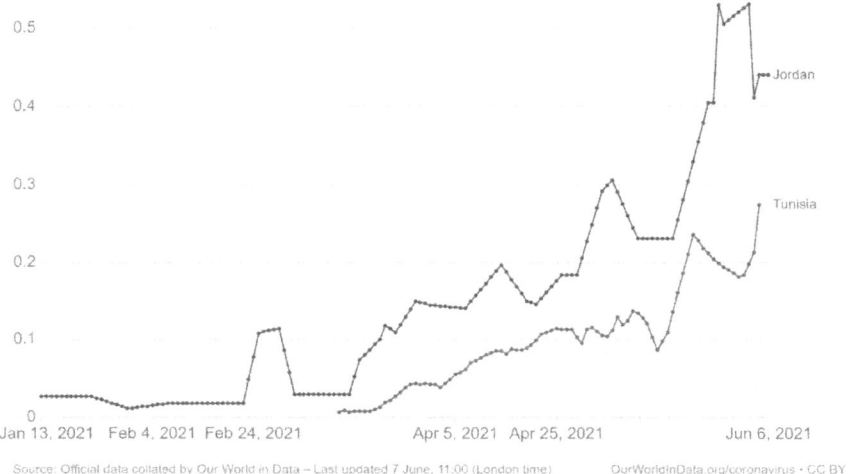

Figure 4.8 Daily COVID-19 vaccine doses administered per 100 people: Jordan and Tunisia

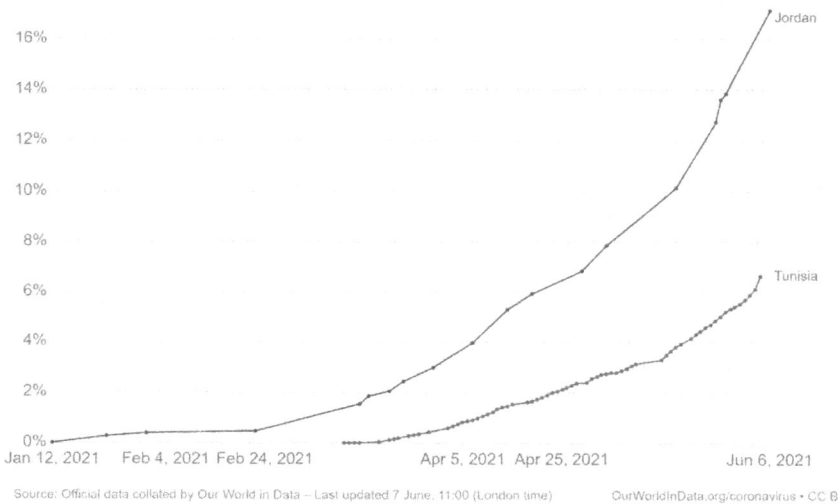

Figure 4.9 Share of people who received at least one dose of COVID-19 vaccine: Jordan and Tunisia

health ministry launched the inoculation program, which provides vaccines free-of-charge to any adult resident in Tunisia provided they registered on the Ministry of Health's online platform. During the first phases, the program prioritized the elderly and high-risk health workers, followed by other health personnel, essential service workers, and people with pre-existing medical conditions.[51] Tunisia so far had set up only 48 vaccination centers across the country but plans to open several others.[52] The country had approved five vaccines (Pfizer/BioNTech, Sputnik V, Johnson & Johnson, Oxford/AstraZeneca, and Sinovac) for use.[53] Then, it announced stopping vaccination with AstraZeneca after the end of the received vaccine doses through COVAX.[54] The national vaccination strategy aims to vaccinate 50% of the adult population by the end of 2021, through the COVAX initiative and doses purchased directly from the manufacturers and supported by the World Bank.[55] However, the vaccination capacities of the country are very limited, especially compared to Jordan, with less than 7% of the population receiving at least one dose of the vaccine by June 4, 2021.[56] In addition to Tunisia's limited health care capacities, there has been some cases of cheating and disorganization in regard to the vaccination strategy, with some people receiving the vaccine before their turn was up and others having to wait for long hours and among crowds to get the jab. Additionally, many Tunisians, including frontline health workers, were skeptical about the vaccine and did not register to get it.[57]

Moving Forward

Although Jordan and Tunisia relatively succeeded in containing the first wave of the coronavirus pandemic, they faced serious economic repercussions following the implemented lockdowns and other restrictions. Already suffering from several structural economic challenges, the two governments had to ease the restrictions and risk a surge in infections in order to limit the economic and social losses. As the new cases started to raise indicating larger second and third waves, several gaps were highlighted. In particular, the public healthcare systems showcased major limitations indicating unpreparedness to face crises and pandemics.

Tunisia, in particular, suffers from several issues including limited medical staff and shortage of medical equipment and intensive care beds, especially in marginalized interior towns. The medical personnel working in public hospitals endures poor working conditions and low pay, which had pushed them to go on a three-day strike in the middle of the pandemic. Altogether, such conditions have negatively affected the services provided to patients. In addition, due to the lack of consistency, with three different governments sworn in in less than a year and three different health ministers holding office since the pandemic started, trust in government had dropped significantly and there have been several protests expressing people's unsatisfaction with the situation. Also, people's support for the implemented restrictions had largely fallen compared to the start of the outbreak and Tunisians showed one of the highest hesitancy rates toward the vaccine.[58] Tunisia needs to reconsider its public healthcare budget and invest in the sector to improve its preparedness for crises. With limited resources and high indebtedness, the country has no choice but to relocate its financing toward such essential sector. Offering targeted subsidies would reduce the overall subsidization budget while privatizing the oversized public companies would eventually ease some of the public debt burden and free some resources. Additionally, the government needs to offer some political stability and assurance, so that the people trust its policies and support it. The country also suffers from a poor governance structure and lacks e-governance and use of digitalization, particularly in the health and education system.[59] Several issues, regarding COVID-19 tracking and vaccine registration, had surfaced, while classes had been often disrupted with no online learning system in place since the start of the outbreak.

Jordan, on the other hand, had performed much better than Tunisia on many levels in terms of its health sector response. However, its public healthcare system also suffers from limited capacity and small budget, which necessitates a relocation of resources to better prepare the system for crisis management. Furthermore, Jordan faces special challenges related to its complex demographic structure, with a large section of refugees unregistered and hence not targeted by foreign aid channels. This calls for a better governance when dealing with refugees and asylum seekers, along with equal response among the different nationalities. In addition, Jordan's particular economic structure, with an overreliance on the service sector, foreign aid, and remittances, makes it significantly exposed to the global shocks associated with the pandemic and the implemented restrictions.[60]

Conclusion

Jordan and Tunisia's initial responses to COVID-19 were considered successful compared to other countries in MENA and elsewhere. Through national lockdowns, the two countries initially contained the outbreak and flattened the first curve by early May 2020. However, these measures had serious economic repercussions, which pushed the two governments toward lifting all restrictions prematurely. This decision, in turn, led to a gradual increase in the daily numbers of new COVID-19 cases. By the fall of 2020, the number of cases and deaths increased significantly indicating much bigger waves in both countries. To control the outbreak, the two countries started their inoculation programs by early 2021, yet they are still short of their initial vaccination targets. To date, Jordan and Tunisia continue to struggle to find the right balance between implementing measures to halt the pandemic and limiting its economic repercussions.

Notes

1 Ben Mimoune, Nejla. Report. *Policy and Institutional Responses to COVID-19 in the Middle East and North Africa: Jordan.* Brookings Doha Center, December 16, 2020. https://www.brookings.edu/research/policy-and-institutional-responses-to-covid-19-in-the-middle-east-and-north-africa-jordan/

Abouzzohour, Yasmina and Nejla Ben Mimoune. Report. *Policy and Institutional Responses to COVID-19 in the Middle East and North Africa: Tunisia.* Brookings Doha Center, December 15, 2020. https://www.brookings.edu/research/policy-and-institutional-responses-to-covid-19-in-the-middle-east-and-north-africa-tunisia/

2 Arraf, Jane. "Jordan keeps coronavirus in check with one of the world's strictest lockdowns." National Public Radio (NPR), March 25, 2020. https://www.npr.org/sections/coronavirus-live-updates/2020/03/25/821349297/jordan-keeps-coronavirus-in-check-with-one-of-world-s-strictest-lockdowns

3 Ritchie, Hannah, Esteban Ortiz-Ospina, Diana Beltekian, Edouard Mathieu, Joe Hasell, Bobbie Macdonald, Charlie Giattino, Cameron Appel, Lucas Rodés-Guirao, and Max Roser. "Jordan and Tunisia: Coronavirus pandemic country profile." Our World in Data. Johns Hopkins University, June 8, 2020. https://ourworldindata.org/coronavirus/country/jordan?country=JOR~TUN

4 Ben Mimoune. *Policy and Institutional Responses to COVID-19 in the Middle East and North Africa: Jordan.*

5 Ritchie et al. "Jordan and Tunisia: Coronavirus pandemic country profile."

Note: The numbers cover the period of March 3, 2020, through May 3, 2020, corresponding to the first wave of COVD-19 in Jordan.

6 Dyer, Paul, Isaac Schaider, and Andrew Letzkus. "Infographic: The incidence of COVID-19 in the Middle East and North Africa." (blog). Brookings Doha Center, December 23, 2020. https://www.brookings.edu/interactives/infographic-the-incidence-of-covid-19-in-the-middle-east-and-north-africa/

7 Ben Mimoune. *Policy and institutional responses to COVID-19 in the Middle East and North Africa: Jordan.*

"The Official Website of the Jordanian Ministry of Health: Coronavirus Disease." Jordan Ministry of Health. Accessed May 28, 2021. https://corona.moh.gov.jo/en

8 Arraf. "Jordan keeps coronavirus in check with one of the world's strictest lockdowns."

9 The indicator addresses formal policy responses and should not be confused with actual effectiveness.

10 Dyer, Paul, Isaac Schaider, and Andrew Letzkus. "Infographic: New COVID-19 cases and the stringency of governmental response in the Middle East and North Africa." (blog). Brookings Doha Center, January 12, 2021. https://www.brookings.edu/interactives/infographic-new-covid-19-cases-and-the-stringency-of-governmental-response-in-the-middle-east-and-north-africa/

11 For more details about institutional response, see Ben Mimoune. *Policy and Institutional Responses to COVID-19 in the Middle East and North Africa: Jordan.*

12 CFR is the ratio of the confirmed deaths to the confirmed cases. This rate gives us an idea about an infection's mortality risk. However, in the case of a pandemic such as COVID-19, this rate is often an overestimation of death risk since often the actual total number of infections/cases is much higher than the confirmed/reported one.

Dyer, Paul, Isaac Schaider, and Andrew Letzkus. "Infographic: COVID-19 fatality in the Middle East and North Africa." (blog). Brookings Doha Center, December 30, 2020. https://www.brookings.edu/interactives/infographic-covid-19-fatality-in-the-middle-east-and-north-africa/

13 "Current health expenditure (% of GDP) - Jordan, Tunisia, Egypt, Arab Rep., Morocco, Lebanon." World Development Indicators. The World Bank. Accessed May 28, 2021. https://data.worldbank.org/indicator/SH.XPD.CHEX. GD.ZS?locations=JO-TN-EG-MA-LB

14 "Current health expenditure per capita, PPP (Current International $) - Jordan, Tunisia, Egypt, Arab Rep., Morocco, Lebanon." World Development Indicators. The World Bank. Accessed May 28, 2021. https://data.worldbank.org/indicator/ SH.XPD.CHEX.PP.CD?locations=JO-TN-EG-MA-LB

15 Ben Mimoune. *Policy and Institutional Responses to COVID-19 in the Middle East and North Africa: Jordan.*

16 Abouzzohour and Ben Mimoune. *Policy and Institutional Responses to COVID-19 in the Middle East and North Africa: Tunisia.*

17 Ritchie et al. "Jordan and Tunisia: Coronavirus pandemic country profile."
   Note: The numbers cover the period of March 4, 2020, through May 4, 2020; corresponding to the first wave of COVD-19 in Tunisia.

18 Dyer et al. "Infographic: The incidence of COVID-19 in the Middle East and North Africa."

19 Abouzzohour and Ben Mimoune. *Policy and Institutional Responses to COVID-19 in the Middle East and North Africa: Tunisia.*
   Note: The previously consulted COVID-19 website (https://covid-19.tn/fr/ tableau-de-bord/) is no longer functional.

20 For more on Tunisia's institutional response to the pandemic, see: Abouzzohour and Ben Mimoune. *Policy and Institutional Responses to COVID-19 in the Middle East and North Africa: Tunisia.*

21 Dyer et al. "Infographic: New COVID-19 cases and the stringency of governmental response in the Middle East and North Africa."

22 Abouzzohour and Ben Mimoune. *Policy and Institutional Responses to COVID-19 in the Middle East and North Africa: Tunisia.*

23 "Current health expenditure (% of GDP) - Jordan, Tunisia, Egypt, Arab Rep., Morocco, Lebanon." World Development Indicators.

24 "Current health expenditure per capita, PPP (Current International $) - Jordan, Tunisia, Egypt, Arab Rep., Morocco, Lebanon." World Development Indicators.

25 Abouzzohour and Ben Mimoune. *Policy and Institutional Responses to COVID-19 in the Middle East and North Africa: Tunisia.*

26 Ben Mimoune. *Policy and Institutional Responses to COVID-19 in the Middle East and North Africa: Jordan.*

27 "Tunisie – Tourisme: Quelle est la place du tourisme dans l'économie nationale? [Tunisia - Tourism: What is the place of tourism in the national economy?]" Klynveld Peat Marwick Goerdeler (KPMG). November 28, 2019. https://home. kpmg/tn/fr/home/insights/2019/11/quelle-est-la-place-du-tourisme.html

28 "Pandemic drives down Tunisia's tourism revenue by 65%." January 7, 2021. https://www.reuters.com/article/tunisia-economy-tourism-idAFL1N2JI0I0

29 "IMF Executive Board concludes 2021 Article IV Consultation with Tunisia." *Press Release No. 21/52.* International Monetary Fund (IMF), February 26, 2021. https://www.imf.org/en/News/Articles/2021/02/26/pr2152-tunisia-imf-executive-board-concludes-2021-article-iv-consultation-with-tunisia

30 IMF. *Statistical Appendix: Regional Economic Outlook: Arising from the Pandemic: Building Forward Better.* IMF, April 2021. https://www.imf.org/-/media/ Files/Publications/REO/MCD-CCA/2021/April/English/statsapp.ashx

31 Ibid.
   "Tunisia and the IMF." IMF. Accessed May 30, 2021. https://www.imf.org/en/ Countries/TUN
   "Jordan and the IMF." IMF. Accessed May 30, 2021. https://www.imf.org/en/ Countries/JOR

"Jordan and the IMF: Frequently asked questions." IMF, December 14, 2020. https://www.imf.org/en/Countries/JOR/FAQ#Q1

32 "Unemployment, total (% of total labor force) (modeled ILO estimate) - Tunisia." World development indicators. The World Bank. Accessed May 30, 2021. https://data.worldbank.org/indicator/SL.UEM.TOTL.ZS?locations=TN

33 The authors estimate the poverty increase to be between 6.5% and 7.3% after the government's interventions targeting those mostly impacted by the pandemic. See Kokas, Deeksha, Gladys Lopez-Acevedo, Abdel Rahman El Lahga, and Vibhuti Mendiratta. "Impacts of COVID-19 on household welfare in Tunisia." World Bank, Policy Research Working Paper 9503. December 2020. https://documents1.worldbank.org/curated/en/529381608228318922/pdf/Impacts-of-COVID-19-on-Household-Welfare-in-Tunisia.pdf

34 For more on government support initiatives, see: Ben Mimoune. *Policy and Institutional Responses to COVID-19 in the Middle East and North Africa: Jordan*, and Abouzzohour and Ben Mimoune. *Policy and Institutional Responses to COVID-19 in the Middle East and North Africa: Tunisia.*

35 Ibid.

36 Ibid.

Abouzzohour, Yasmina. "One year of COVID-19 in the Middle East and North Africa: The fate of the 'best performers.'" *Order from Chaos* (blog). Brookings, March 22, 2021. https://www.brookings.edu/blog/order-from-chaos/2021/03/22/one-year-of-covid-19-in-the-middle-east-and-north-africa-the-fate-of-the-best-performers/

37 *Pandemic Fatigue Reinvigorating the Public to Prevent COVID-19.* World Health Organization (WHO) Regional Office for Europe, 2020. https://apps.who.int/iris/bitstream/handle/10665/335820/WHO-EURO-2020-1160-40906–55390-eng.pdf

38 "Opinion leaders, national sample see gov't as 'successful' in limiting COVID-19 — poll." *The Jordan Times*, June 24, 2020. https://www.jordan-times.com/news/local/opinion-leaders-national-sample-see-govt-%E2%80%98successful%E2%80%99-limiting-covid-19-%E2%80%94-poll

39 Al-Shami, Salma. "Citizens weigh in on the health of their healthcare systems in MENA." Arab Barometer, April 7, 2021. https://www.arabbarometer.org/2021/04/citizens-weigh-in-on-the-health-of-their-healthcare-systems-in-mena/

40 "Etude et résultats sur l'état du tunisien sous confinement réalisée en Avril 2020 [Study and results on the state of the Tunisian under confinement carried out in April 2020]." Sigma Conseil, April 6, 2020. http://www.sigma.tn/Fr/actualites_7_10_D86

41 Al-Shami. "Citizens weigh in on the health of their healthcare systems in MENA."

42 "Tunisian hospitals buckle under COVID crisis." *Reuters*, April 28, 2021. https://www.reuters.com/world/africa/tunisian-hospitals-buckle-under-covid-crisis-2021–04–28/

43 Abouzzohour and Ben Mimoune. *Policy and Institutional Responses to COVID-19 in the Middle East and North Africa: Tunisia.*

44 "Covid: Jordan's health minister quits over hospital oxygen deaths." *BBC News*, March 13, 2021. https://www.bbc.com/news/world-middle-east-56381870

45 Al-Shami. "Citizens weigh in on the health of their healthcare systems in MENA."

46 "Jordan's coronavirus vaccination programme to start next week – minister." *Reuters*. January 9, 2021. https://www.reuters.com/article/health-coronavirus-vaccination-jordan-in-idUSKBN29E0MF

"COVID-19 Vaccine." UNHCR Jordan. Accessed June 8, 2021. https://help.unhcr.org/jordan/en/frequently-asked-questions-unhcr/covid-19-vaccine/

47 "Jordan." COVID19 vaccine tracker. Accessed June 8, 2021. https://covid19.
    trackvaccines.org/country/jordan/
48 "Jordan to receive 10.2 million doses of coronavirus vaccines this year." *Arab-
    News*. March 19, 2021. https://arab.news/9teq5
49 "Jordan's coronavirus vaccination programme to start next week – minister."
    Reuters. Al Sherbini, Ramadan. "COVID-19: Jordan aims to administer 3 million
    doses by June for 'safe summer'." *GulfNews*. April 9, 2021. https://gulfnews.com/
    world/mena/covid-19-jordan-aims-to-administer-3-million-doses-by-june-for-
    safe-summer-1.78466362
50 Ritchie et al. "COVID-19 vaccine doses administered: Jordan and Tunisia." Our
    World in Data. Johns Hopkins University. Accessed June 8, 2021. https://our-
    worldindata.org/grapher/cumulative-covid-vaccinations?country=JOR~TUN
51 Marouane, Leila. "Tunisia receives first batch of COVID-19 vaccines through
    COVAX facility." ReliefWeb. News and Press Release from the World
    Health Organization. March 17, 2021. https://reliefweb.int/report/tunisia/
    tunisia-receives-first-batch-covid-19-vaccines-through-covax-facility
    "World Bank approves US$100 million to support COVID-19 vaccine de-
    ployment in Tunisia." World Bank. Press Release. March 26, 2021. https://
    www.worldbank.org/en/news/press-release/2021/03/26/world-bank-approves-us-
    100-million-to-support-covid-19-vaccine-deployment-in-tunisia
52 "Covid-19: Neuf nouveaux centre de vaccination [Covid-19: Nine new
    vaccination centers]." *MosaiqueFM*. April 27, 2021. https://www.mosaiquefm.
    net/fr/actualite-national-tunisie/889628/covid-19-neuf-nouveaux-centre-de-
    vaccination
53 "Tunisia." COVID19 Vaccine Tracker. Accessed June 8, 2021. https://covid19.
    trackvaccines.org/country/Tunisia/
54 "Stopping the vaccination with "AstraZeneca" after the end of the vaccine
    doses." *MosaiqueFM*. June 4, 2021. https://bit.ly/3pB1K41
55 "World Bank approves US$100 million to support COVID-19 vaccine deploy-
    ment in Tunisia." World Bank.
56 Ritchie et al. "COVID-19 vaccine doses administered: Jordan and Tunisia."
57 Ben Mbarek, Ghaya. "Tunisia. Anti-Vax Hospital Workers and Line Jumpers Com-
    plicate Vaccine Rollout." Nawaat. April 14, 2021. https://nawaat.org/2021/04/14/
    tunisia-anti-vax-hospital-workers-and-line-jumpers-complicate-vaccine-rollout/
58 Schaer, Cathrin and Kersten Knipp. "Tunisia's third COVID-19 wave: Doctors
    warn of health system collapse." *Deutsche Welle (DW)*. May 4, 2021. https://www.
    dw.com/en/tunisia-covid-19-doctors-warn-of-health-system-collapse/a-57425281
59 Guetat, Meriem. "Tunisia and coronavirus: The reality of a poor governance." Ital-
    ian Institute for International Political Studies (ISPI), Commentary. April 9, 2020.
    https://www.ispionline.it/it/pubblicazione/tunisia-and-coronavirus-reality-
    poor-governance-25671
60 Singh, Manjari. "Jordan after COVID-19: From crisis adjustment to crisis man-
    agement." Washington Institute, Fikra Forum Policy Analysis. April 15, 2020.
    https://www.washingtoninstitute.org/policy-analysis/jordan-after-covid-19-
    crisis-adjustment-crisis-management

References

Abouzzohour, Yasmina. "One year of COVID-19 in the Middle East and North Africa:
    The fate of the 'best performers.'" *Order from Chaos* (blog). Brookings, March 22,
    2021. https://www.brookings.edu/blog/order-from-chaos/2021/03/22/one-year-of-
    covid-19-in-the-middle-east-and-north-africa-the-fate-of-the-best-performers/

Abouzzohour, Yasmina and Nejla Ben Mimoune. Report. *Policy and Institutional Responses to COVID-19 in the Middle East and North Africa: Tunisia.* Brookings Doha Center, December 15, 2020. https://www.brookings.edu/research/policy-and-institutional-responses-to-covid-19-in-the-middle-east-and-north-africa-tunisia/

Al-Shami, Salma. "Citizens weigh in on the health of their healthcare systems in MENA." Arab Barometer, April 7, 2021. https://www.arabbarometer.org/2021/04/citizens-weigh-in-on-the-health-of-their-healthcare-systems-in-mena/

Arraf, Jane. "Jordan keeps coronavirus in check with one of the world's strictest lockdowns." National Public Radio (NPR), March 25, 2020. https://www.npr.org/sections/coronavirus-live-updates/2020/03/25/821349297/jordan-keeps-coronavirus-in-check-with-one-of-world-s-strictest-lockdowns

Ben Mimoune, Nejla. Report. *Policy and Institutional Responses to COVID-19 in the Middle East and North Africa: Jordan.* Brookings Doha Center, December 16, 2020. https://www.brookings.edu/research/policy-and-institutional-responses-to-covid-19-in-the-middle-east-and-north-africa-jordan/

"Covid: Jordan's health minister quits over hospital oxygen deaths." *BBC News*, March 13, 2021. https://www.bbc.com/news/world-middle-east-56381870

"COVID-19 vaccine." UNHCR Jordan. Accessed June 8, 2021. https://help.unhcr.org/jordan/en/frequently-asked-questions-unhcr/covid-19-vaccine/.

Dyer, Paul, Isaac Schaider, and Andrew Letzkus. "Infographic: COVID-19 fatality in the Middle East and North Africa." (blog). Brookings Doha Center, December 30, 2020. https://www.brookings.edu/interactives/infographic-covid-19-fatality-in-the-middle-east-and-north-africa/

Dyer, Paul, Isaac Schaider, and Andrew Letzkus. "Infographic: New COVID-19 cases and the stringency of governmental response in the Middle East and North Africa." (blog). Brookings Doha Center, January 12, 2021. https://www.brookings.edu/interactives/infographic-new-covid-19-cases-and-the-stringency-of-governmental-response-in-the-middle-east-and-north-africa/

Dyer, Paul, Isaac Schaider, and Andrew Letzkus. "Infographic: The incidence of COVID-19 in the Middle East and North Africa." (blog). Brookings Doha Center, December 23, 2020. https://www.brookings.edu/interactives/infographic-the-incidence-of-covid-19-in-the-middle-east-and-north-africa/

"Etude et résultats sur l'état du tunisien sous confinement réalisée en Avril 2020 [Study and results on the state of the Tunisian under confinement carried out in April 2020]." Sigma Conseil, April 6, 2020. http://www.sigma.tn/Fr/actualites_7_10_D86.

IMF. *Statistical Appendix: Regional Economic Outlook: Arising from the Pandemic: Building Forward Better.* IMF, April 2021. https://www.imf.org/-/media/Files/Publications/REO/MCD-CCA/2021/April/English/statsapp.ashx

"IMF Executive Board Concludes 2021 Article IV Consultation with Tunisia." *Press Release No. 21/52.* International Monetary Fund (IMF), February 26, 2021. https://www.imf.org/en/News/Articles/2021/02/26/pr2152-tunisia-imf-executive-board-concludes-2021-article-iv-consultation-with-tunisia.

"Jordan." COVID19 vaccine tracker. Accessed June 8, 2021. https://covid19.trackvaccines.org/country/jordan/

"Jordan and the IMF." IMF. Accessed May 30, 2021. https://www.imf.org/en/Countries/JOR

"Jordan and the IMF: Frequently asked questions." IMF, December 14, 2020. https://www.imf.org/en/Countries/JOR/FAQ#Q1

"Jordan to receive 10.2 million doses of coronavirus vaccines this year." *ArabNews*. March 19, 2021. https://arab.news/9teq5

"Jordan's coronavirus vaccination programme to start next week – minister." *Reuters*. Al Sherbini, Ramadan. "COVID-19: Jordan aims to administer 3 million doses by June for 'safe summer'." *GulfNews*. April 9, 2021. https://gulfnews.com/world/mena/covid-19-jordan-aims-to-administer-3-million-doses-by-june-for-safe-summer-1.78466362

Kokas, Deeksha, Gladys Lopez-Acevedo, Abdel Rahman El Lahga, and Vibhuti Mendiratta. "Impacts of COVID-19 on household welfare in Tunisia." World Bank, Policy Research Working Paper 9503. December 2020. https://documents1.worldbank.org/curated/en/529381608228318922/pdf/Impacts-of-COVID-19-on-Household-Welfare-in-Tunisia.pdf

Marouane, Leila. "Tunisia receives first batch of COVID-19 vaccines through COVAX Facility." ReliefWeb. News and Press Release from the World Health Organization. March 17, 2021. https://reliefweb.int/report/tunisia/tunisia-receives-first-batch-covid-19-vaccines-through-covax-facility

"Opinion leaders, national sample see gov't as 'successful' in limiting COVID-19 — Poll." *The Jordan Times*, June 24, 2020. https://www.jordantimes.com/news/local/opinion-leaders-national-sample-see-govt-%E2%80%98success-ful%E2%80%99-limiting-covid-19-%E2%80%94-poll

"Pandemic drives down Tunisia's Tourism revenue by 65%." January 7, 2021. https://www.reuters.com/article/tunisia-economy-tourism-idAFL1N2JI0I0

Pandemic Fatigue Reinvigorating the Public to Prevent COVID-19. World Health Organization (WHO) Regional Office for Europe, 2020. https://apps.who.int/iris/bitstream/handle/10665/335820/WHO-EURO-2020-1160-40906-55390-eng.pdf

Ritchie, Hannah, Esteban Ortiz-Ospina, Diana Beltekian, Edouard Mathieu, Joe Hasell, Bobbie Macdonald, Charlie Giattino, Cameron Appel, Lucas Rodés-Guirao, and Max Roser. "Jordan: Coronavirus pandemic country profile." Our World in Data. Johns Hopkins University, May 23, 2021. https://ourworldindata.org/coronavirus/country/jordan?country=JOR~TUN

"Tunisian hospitals buckle under COVID crisis." *Reuters*, April 28, 2021. https://www.reuters.com/world/africa/tunisian-hospitals-buckle-under-covid-crisis-2021-04-28/.

"Tunisie – Tourisme: Quelle est la place du tourisme dans l'économie nationale? [Tunisia - Tourism: What is the place of tourism in the national economy?]" Klynveld Peat Marwick Goerdeler (KPMG). November 28, 2019. https://home.kpmg/tn/fr/home/insights/2019/11/quelle-est-la-place-du-tourisme.html

"World Bank approves US$100 million to support COVID-19 Vaccine Deployment in Tunisia." World Bank. Press Release. March 26, 2021. https://www.worldbank.org/en/news/press-release/2021/03/26/world-bank-approves-us-100-million-to-support-covid-19-vaccine-deployment-in-tunisia

World Development Indicators Database. The World Bank. Accessed May 28, 2021. https://data.worldbank.org/indicator/SH.XPD.CHEX.PP.CD?locations=JO-TN-EG-MA-LB.

5 Resilient Authoritarianism and Global Pandemics

Egypt after COVID-19

Lucia Ardovini

Introduction

The outbreak of COVID-19 and its quick spread across the Middle East and North Africa (MENA) region shone a light on the unpreparedness of states and societies that, long before the pandemic, were already struggling to cope with the effects of decades of social unrest, failing state institutions, interrupted political transitions, civil wars and proxy conflicts. In turn, different state reactions to COVID-19 exposed glaring differences in state capacity and economic resources. Nevertheless, a common response to the pandemic has been its securitization. As different countries imposed states of emergency and rulers seized extra-constitutional powers to enforce lockdowns and limit social gatherings, a clear takeaway is that the securitization of the pandemic is resulting into the tightening of authoritarian measures and of state control over society. These extraordinary measures are unlikely to be lifted once the health threat is under control, leading many to speculate that several states across the region are using COVID-19 as a smokescreen to trial new modalities of repression against social and political mobilization.

This chapter analyses the impact that the outbreak of COVID-19 has had on Egyptian society and institutions, focusing on the way in which state responses to the pandemics shed light on ongoing attempts to further institutionalize authoritarianism in the country. Egypt was in a deep state of unrest even before the outbreak of the epidemic, which saw the counter-revolution perpetrated by the military regime of President Abdel Fattah el-Sisi cracking down on dissent and civil liberties, consequently leading to growing manifestations of discontent and worsening popular grievances. Since March 2020, the country's deep-seated issues such as widespread corruption, social inequalities and systemic poverty have only worsened as a consequence of the inadequate response to COVID-19, further threatening the already fading legitimacy of the regime. The reality and urgency of these challenges have led the Egyptian regime to prioritize controlling the narrative around the pandemic over fighting the spread of the virus itself – a task that was simplified by the already authoritarian measures ruling over the country. Yet, the regime's attempts to shift the attention away from the

DOI: 10.4324/9781003266259-5

reality of the threat by accusing its political opponents of misinformation and further cracking down on media and freedom of speech have wielded the opposite results and rather generated renewed attention to the inadequacy of state institutions. From this, the chapter focuses on the regime's responses to COVID-19 to track the drastic impact that the virus is having on the country's already fragile economy and ongoing social issues. It shows that the discontent generated by the regime's inadequate response to COVID-19 is having a direct impact on patterns of social transformation and unrest in the country, possibly dealing an unprecedented blow to resilient authoritarianism.

The chapter first focuses on resilient authoritarianism in Egypt, offering an overview of the intertwining factors that are at the core of the country's historical lack of political space. In particular, it highlights how the almost uninterrupted rule of a state of emergency and the military's deep-seated role within state institutions are two elements that are key to President el-Sisi's counter-revolutionary regime. From this, the securitization process that drives repressive measures and emergency legislations in the country has also shaped regime responses to the COVID-19 pandemic, leading to further crackdown on freedom of expression, assembly and on the already limited political space. Having provided a background on resilient authoritarianism in Egypt, the chapter then moves onto the analysis of state responses to COVID-19 and highlights how, once again, emergency measures meant to deal with the pandemic are instead mostly targeting political opposition to the military regime. Overall, this shows that there are deep cracks in el-Sisi's strongman façade and that the crisis brought about by the pandemic is exacerbating pre-existing structural issues in the country, further eroding the legitimacy of the regime.

Resilient Authoritarianism

Almost ten years after the popular uprisings that briefly subverted the *status quo*, overthrowing the rule of long-standing dictator Hosni Mubarak and opening up the political space to previously suppressed actors and movements, Egypt is back to square one. The military *coup d'etat* that violently removed the country's first democratically elected president, Mohammad Morsi, from power not only posed a symbolic end to the dreams at the core of the Arab uprisings but also marked the beginning of counter-revolutionary rule. Under president and military strongman, el–Sisi's Egypt is undergoing a counter-revolution that completely swept away what was achieved after the democratic revolts, making room for yet another military autocracy to take over the country. Seven years on, Egypt is in the midst of the worst human rights crisis of its troubled history, poverty levels are ramping up and state institutions are proving incapable to cope with the social, economic and political crisis brought about by COVID-19. If anything, the spread of the pandemic is further highlighting Egypt's deep-seated structural issue, reigniting popular discontent and fading levels of popular trust in the military regime. In such an unstable context, el-Sisi has reacted by doing what he knows best: escalating authoritarian measures and tightening even more the already suffocating state control over society. Yet, while the seizing of extra-constitutional powers has long become a paradigm of rule in Egypt, the way in which the regime is mishandling the pandemic reveals that, despite his strongman appearance, the foundations of el-Sisi's power are more fragile than what he wants to let on.

There is a broad body of literature that focuses on the resilience of authoritarianism in Egypt, both before and after the Arab uprisings. In recent years, a growing number of scholars have sought to engage with questions about political transition across Egypt, especially questioning the longevity of the democratic reforms introduced after Mubarak's removal. Neil Ketchley, Cherif Bassiouni, Carrie R. Wickham and Marina Ottaway, among others, have offered explanations for the lack of stability that has come to characterize the country, pointing to seminal issues such as the pervasive role of the military forces within state institutions, a fragile economy, lack of democratic practices and the permanence of emergency laws.[1] Combined, all these elements are at the core of resilient authoritarianism in the country, with emergency laws and securitization techniques being at the heart of el-Sisi's military regime.

Applying a securitization lens to the understanding of resilient authoritarianism in Egypt is key to understanding the extent to which rule by extra-constitutional powers has become a synonym for governance in the country. Nicola Pratt and Dina Rezk offer a clear unpacking of how securitization theories can be applied to non-Western and non-democratic contexts, particularly showing how in the case of Egypt securitization processes have been fundamental to normalizing and institutionalizing state violence and repression.[2] A coercive apparatus that relies on widespread power of control and surveillance, combined with an almost permanent state of emergency, partially explains the resilience of Egyptian authoritarianism but repression alone cannot sustain autocratic rule over a number of decades. Rather, referring to Gramsci's concept of hegemony, Pratt and Rezk maintain that "any dominant class exercises power not only through mechanisms of coercion, such as the police, military and the legal system but also through consent, using a variety of non-coercive means including political institutions, economic/material benefits and culture".[3] In the case of Egypt, this has taken the form of an "authoritarian bargain" between the ruler and the ruled, where various regimes historically derived legitimacy by portraying themselves as the "guarantors of Egyptian sovereignty and progress against both internal and external threats".[4] It follows that regime repression is dependent upon winning consent among citizens against a perceived threat, with opposition movements such as the Muslim Brotherhood historically being the main target of state violence.

Yet, the escalation of police brutality and indiscriminate arrests in the decade leading up to the 2011 Uprisings largely upset the hegemonic balance, which also suffered from the economic crisis that saw the cut of social and economic benefits. The restrictions on political space and civil rights imposed by the almost permanent state of emergency were not enough to keep popular grievances under control, rather, the state of emergency itself became one of the main issues driving the outbreak of the uprisings. Egyptian authoritarianism is in fact characterized by the co-dependent relationship between governance and emergency legislations, referring to a legal construct that originates from multiple constitutional articles, amendments, decrees, and legislations that collectively grant the executive extensive extra-constitutional discretionary powers.[5] Emergency laws blur the lines between military and civilian legal processes, as well as facilitating the restriction of civil liberties and expanding police and military powers. The cyclical imposition of emergency legislations has long become the dominant paradigm of government in the country, dating back to its first application in 1922. From then, the seemingly unbreakable link between governance and emergency legislations went on to characterize the rule of Gamal Nasser, Anwar Sadat and Hosni Mubarak, who all relied on extra-constitutional powers to derogate from the rule of law and resort to repressive measures to maintain their fading legitimacy.[6]

Emergency legislations were briefly lifted between May 1980 and October 1981, until they expired in June 2012. This exception did not last long, however, as the Morsi government re-introduced emergency law in January 2013. Shortly thereafter, following his removal by the military forces and the August 2013 Rabaa and Nahda Square massacres, the interim government re-introduced a state of emergency that was routinely briefly suspended and then imposed again until April 2017, when el-Sisi imposed a new state of emergency following attacks on two Coptic churches.[7] Emergency legislations have been routinely renewed since then and remain in place at the time of writing. These new regulations and amendments to the legal code are allowing the el–Sisi's regime to widen the sphere of repression beyond the Muslim Brotherhood, targeting anyone who expresses dissent against the regime, particularly zoning in on human rights organizations and journalist and even including many of those who supported the *coup* against Morsi. This is made possible by the 2014 anti-terrorism law that includes in its scope any "act" that might obstruct the work of public officials, institutions and so on, prescribes a prison sentence of up to 10 years for anyone who is part of a group that "harms national unity or social peace" while also allowing for the military trial of civilians.[8] Since then, additional amendments and laws outlaw protests and gatherings without a permit, censor independent media and severely curtail the activities of non-governmental organizations. As a result, the number of indiscriminate arrests has skyrocketed along with that of enforced disappearances, with 17 new prisons being built to accommodate the unprecedented number of prisoners.[9] el-Sisi justifies these draconian measures by claiming that they are in place to "protect the people" from terrorism and international threats, but what they effectively lead to is the development of a narrative that portrays Egypt as being in a permanent state of emergency. What has changed, however, is that the complete annihilation of political space and rampant human rights abuses are leading to growing popular dissatisfaction despite the harsh crackdown on dissent, which reveal the existence of deep cracks in the military regime.

It therefore does not come as a surprise that, in such a fragile context, the regime's immediate response to the COVID-19 pandemic was first to deny it and then to immediately securitize the health threat. If anything, the outbreak of the pandemic provided the regime with yet another excuse to seize even more extra-constitutional powers. Emergency Law has been amended to specifically address the pandemic, however, only 5 of the 18 proposed amendments are clearly tied to public health developments, demonstrating that the focus is more on entrenching repression than tackling the virus.[10] The amendments grant the president greater powers to deal with the health crisis, but also further suffocate dissent by suspending universities and schools, imposing a night-time curfew and by granting both the police and the military forces the power of banning assemblies without reference to public health reasons.[11] Indeed, the resort to framing the pandemic as a threat to "national security and public order" reflects the security mentality that governs Sisi's Egypt. Nevertheless, these heightened repressive measures are failing to contain rising popular discontent and small-scale protests have begun to routinely take place across the country despite the harsh measures in place. As this phenomenon keeps on gaining momentum and criticism against the regime grows on social media and international media channels, it is becoming increasingly clear that COVID-19 is threatening the Egyptian military's perceived hold on society. In turn, this goes against the perception of Egypt's resilient authoritarianism as impossible to dismantle and questions the application of the "authoritarian-persistence" literature to this particular case, as it equates the longevity of regimes in the region with an assumed stability of their political orders.[12] If anything, the wide socio-political and economic crisis brought about by the pandemic shows that, in el-Sisi's Egypt, it does not seem to be the case.

COVID-19 and Regime Responses

The spread of COVID-19 to Egypt poses a serious threat to the stability of the regime. Since the 2013 *coup d'etat*, military rule has not only wiped out what little gains were made after the 2011 uprisings but has also driven Egypt into the worst human rights crisis of its history. A renewed wave of popular uprisings in the last few months of 2019 revealed that the country's deep-seated issues, such as widespread corruption, social inequalities and systemic poverty remain a key driver of popular discontent.[13] The reality and urgency of these challenges have led the Egyptian government to prioritize controlling the narrative over fighting the spread of the virus itself – with potentially disastrous results. The weakness and unpreparedness of much of the Egyptian state, complicated by the ever-growing role of the military, makes the challenge even more acute.

Egypt appears to be the among the worst-hit North African countries by the COVID-19 pandemic so far, with over 114,000 confirmed cases at the time of writing and the widespread belief that the real numbers are indeed drastically higher, despite the regime's attempts to disguise the number of infections.[14] The country's burgeoning population of over 100 million people features the perfect structural conditions for a virus to spread exponentially fast, and other demographic data only add to this worrying picture. It is estimated that Egyptians live on approximately only 5% of the land, making it almost impossible to practice any form of social distancing.[15] Moreover, an estimated 35% of Egyptians live below the poverty line, meaning that many are reliant on day-to-day business and trade to get by, with their livelihoods being considerably threatened by the imposition of security measures such as curfew and limitations on freedoms of movement. The first confirmed cases of COVID-19 were reported in the tourist city of Luxor on February 14, 2020, with numbers escalating exponentially from then on. From the very beginning, the regime attempted to cover up the number of infections and refused to carry out tests so as not scare tourists away at the very peak of the tourist season, especially as the sector had just started to recover from the turmoil that followed the 2011 uprisings.[16] Egypt's economy is heavily dependent on the tourism industry, as are thousands of locals and workers from across the country who flock to tourist hotspots for seasonal work. To put things into perspective, in 2018–2019 alone, 11,346,000 people traveled to Egypt generating approximately 12.6 million US dollars.[17] Nevertheless, as the virus continued to spread, officials were forced to shut down all airports on March 16, essentially putting an end to a season that had just begun. While it is too early to speculate, economists estimate that the loss of income from tourism could reach $1 billion per month if these measures remain in place, which for now they undoubtedly will.[18]

The first measurable impact of the pandemic in the country is therefore the blow that is already dealing with Egypt's fragile economy, which heavily relies on external funding and tourism revenues. Once the reality of the threat could not be disguised anymore, the regime acted quickly, implementing various measures to curb the spread of the virus such as travel bans, a night-time curfew enforced by police patrols from 8 p.m. to 6 a.m., bans on gathering and the closure of schools, universities and religious institutions.[19] Nevertheless, despite the regime's attempt to strike a balance between health concerns and economic considerations, the partial lockdown is causing significant disruptions and having a negative effect on the economic progress that Egypt achieved over the past couple of years. The government is attempting to support economic activities via accommodating fiscal and monetary policies, such as allocating 100 billion Egyptian Pounds (EGP) to combat some of the economic fallout from COVID-19, cutting interest rates, providing loans with reduced interest rates to support the hardest hit sectors and expanding social safety nets.[20] Nevertheless, these efforts are proving unsuccessful and the quickly sinking economy, combined with widespread corruption and widening social inequalities, mean that the unemployed and the working classes will be those who get hit the hardest, further contributing to the growth of popular grievances and discontent.

Fighting the Virus, Hiding the Cracks

Concerns over the economic fallout of the pandemic might therefore explain the first reaction of the regime, which initially attempt to mostly discredit the gravity of the health threat. In particular, a mock interview with a character wearing grotesque green face mask studded with spikes to mimic the coronavirus cell conducted on al-Hayah, a popular commercial channel, went viral, with the coronavirus complaints of "unjust treatment" because of widespread "exaggeration", accusing social media of hyping the epidemic's severity and calling on viewers to follow basic hygiene rules.[21] From this, one can also argue that the regime's awareness of their unpreparedness to deal with a threat of this kind also played a considerable part in the way in which the pandemic is being handled, overall revealing that there are deep cracks in el-Sisi's strongman façade.

The regime's attempt to downplay the scale of the threat posed by the pandemic can indeed be attributed to structural challenges and insecurities, yet the speed at which the virus continues to spread and its impact on socio, political and economic issues considerably complicate such a task. Nevertheless, it is not surprising that the regime in Egypt seems more concerned about silencing those who denounce the virus's impact on the country's fragile society rather than effectively trying to fight the disease itself.[22] This is due to one of the biggest challenges to el-Sisi's legitimacy, which is the fading levels of popular support – or even tolerance – for the military rule. Almost one year after the outbreak of the pandemic, it is becoming increasingly clear that, globally, virus containment and management measures are more effective when populations trust their government; however, the military regime has long lacked transparency and inspires fear rather than trust. An added layer is the fact that the majority of Egypt's population has only ever known life under emergency legislations and therefore associates political rule with the seizing of extra-constitutional powers. While the embeddedness of such draconian rules within state institutions facilitate the imposition of curfews and lockdown, the securitization of the pandemic has led to escalating emergency measures that are resulting in the potential for increased repression. In such a context, a real societal concern is that the regime's tightened control over freedom of expression and assembly will not be lifted once the COVID-19 crisis is over.

The imposition of lockdown measures and the strengthening of emergency rule in response to the pandemic is not necessarily a challenge in itself, as Egypt existed under a state of emergency for the majority of its history as a nation state. Rather, what is proving to be challenging is doing so without lowering the population trust's in institutions even more. The denial and misinformation propagated by state-owned media during the outbreak of the pandemic generated a widespread distrust towards the regime's approach to the seriousness of the virus. In addition to official narratives claiming that Egypt is "untouchable" and the Egyptians "are immune to coronavirus", several public figures also further dismissed the gravity of the threat while various conspiracy theories quickly gained momentum on social media.[23] Yet, once the scale of the pandemic could not be dismissed anymore, the regime resorted to cracking down even more on freedom of expression and by accusing its political opponents of spreading misinformation. Such an approach in itself is also not new, as resilient authoritarianism greatly depends on restrictions on independent media and voices, but it appears that under the new emergency legislations el-Sisi is taking this even further.

Perhaps unsurprisingly, in the bid to shift the attention away from the reality of the COVID crisis, one of the first responses was to point the finger at the banned Muslim Brotherhood, accusing the Islamist organization of spreading panic and fear by reporting fake statistics of infection.[24] What is more concerning is the further crackdown on political and human rights activists, as seen by the arrest on March 19 of four prominent activists – Mona Seif, Laila Soueif, Ahdaf Soueif and Rabab al-Mahdi – who staged a public protest to raise concerns about the potential spread of the virus in Egypt's infamously overcrowded prisons.[25] Similarly, British journalists Ruth Michaelson, who works for the Guardian, had their press credentials revoked and were banned from the country after reporting that, based on a study by the University of Toronto, the number of cases of COVID-19 in Egypt in March 2020 was likely closer to 19,000 rather than the reported 456.[26] While this does not necessarily come as a surprise, given Egypt's crackdown on journalism and free speech, it is deeply concerning that censorship remains in place despite the spread of a potentially crippling pandemic.[27]

Ongoing Crisis

Overall, the securitization of the COVID-19 pandemic has provided another excuse for the Egyptian regime to expand its powers and crackdown on rights, freedoms and rule of law in the country. The pandemic is definitely threatening the Egyptian military's perceived hold on society, resulting in the escalation of the regime's hard-handed approaches to keep civilians in line. In ways reminiscent to the post-coup events in 2013, the military today is merging anti-COVID-19 measures with reactive brutality and human rights abuse.[28] However, while the way in which the Sisi regime is responding to the spread of the virus is in line with decades of abuse of extra-constitutional powers, systemic inequalities and routine crackdowns on freedom of speech and opposition, the attention that these measures are generating is putting the country back on the international stage. The recent arrest of the head and staff of the Egyptian Initiative for Personal Rights and their subsequent charging with terrorism accusations have sparked international criticism, which could, in turn, affect the country's policy relations with international powers. In particular, the incoming administration of Joe Biden is likely to drastically reshape the relationship between the two countries, which currently see Egypt as being the second biggest received of US monetary and military aid in the region after Israel, estimated at $1.38bn per year.[29] In response to growing concerns over the human rights situation in Egypt, Biden has famously previously stated that "there will be no more blank checks for [Donald] Trump's favourite dictator" which, if followed through, would have a negative impact on both Egypt's diplomatic relations and its domestic economy.[30]

On the domestic level, the way in which the regime is handling the pandemic also reveals that there are some detectable changes in the balance of power typical of Egyptian institutions. In particular, the overt lack of transparency displayed by the Egyptian regime reveals that its institutions are largely unprepared to deal with the crisis, while the ongoing crackdown on information suggests that the president is deeply worried about its decreasing rates of legitimacy. As online opposition movements declare that "Sisi and the coronavirus are two sides of the same danger", the way in which COVID-19 continues on developing will have an even more drastic impact on an already fragile economy and ongoing socio-political issues, possibly dealing an unprecedented blow to resilient authoritarianism.[31] Indeed, some structural changes are already visible, especially in regard to the role of the military within political institutions. The military forces have historically been at the forefront of Egyptian governance and even more so in the aftermath of the 2011 uprisings. The el–Sisi's regime in itself represents a departure from Egypt's military past as while pre-2011 regimes were military in nature, the military as an institution never ruled directly.[32] With el-Sisi in charge the armed forces have enjoyed a much stronger presence, also becoming the "public face" of political institutions in the country.

Yet, while the military immediately stepped forward to respond to the pandemic, it soon became clear that they were not equipped to deal with such crisis. Rather, as Nathan Brown and Amr Hamzawy point out, the regime allowed

> much of the civilian structures of the Egyptian government to set policy within their respective realms. The Ministry of Health provided medical guidance; the Ministry of Education adjusted school hours, testing, and pedagogy; the official religious establishment provided more leadership; and leading civilian officials provided information – including the public health advisor to the president and to the citizenry and imposed a series of restrictions on public life in the name of public health.[33]

There are several reasons behind this shift, most of all the fact that the scope of the required responses clearly exceeds military resources and expertise. Therefore, the pandemic is gradually leading to a new phase of Egyptian governance, one in which civilian bodies have a more direct role in making and implementing policy and, while the military forces are part of the process, their public role in facing the pandemic is quite limited. While it is too early to say whether or not this shift marks a real change for the future of resilient authoritarianism in the country, its relevance should not be dismissed. The clear message to be learnt in this case is that, as Egypt faces an unprecedented challenge, it is its civil society that leads the way forward rather than the military regime.

Conclusion

The responses against COVID-19 staged by Egypt's military regime are consistent with el-Sisi's modality of rule and mostly focused on the securitization of the pandemic in order to further crackdown on freedom of speech and civil rights. Securitization processes and the routine imposition of emergency legislations have been at the very heart of Egypt's resilient authoritarianism, yet, failing responses to the pandemic reveal that the regime's stability might indeed be under threat. Escalating attempts to further crackdown on independent media and human rights activists – as seen in the recent case of the arrest of the head and staff of the Egyptian Initiative for Personal Rights – also further support this argument, as the regime keeps on descending into the frenzied pursuit of perceived threats with unprecedented amount of violence. While this is not necessarily new, el-Sisi's frantic attempts to hold onto legitimacy have started to have both domestic and international repercussions. On the international level, escalating and blatant abuses of human rights meant that European powers cannot ignore regime brutality anymore, despite trade relations with the country and their support for Egypt's role in controlling migration flows and its ongoing involvement in Libya.[34] Domestically, while the regime's responses to the pandemic appear irrational and exaggerated, they also betray its preoccupation over simmering popular discontent and dissent. The structural issues at the heart of the 2011 uprisings, such as corruption, social inequalities, escalating levels of poverty and the lack of political space have not been addressed, rather, the situation has worsened under the counter-revolutionary regime. Egypt does not exist in a vacuum and is therefore affected by the ongoing social transformations happening elsewhere in the MENA region, as well has having a very young population that vividly remembers their involvement in the 2011 uprisings that briefly challenged the status quo in the country. The ongoing crackdown on dissent therefore demonstrates that the regime is also incredibly aware of growing discontent and of its fading legitimacy, which is desperately trying to reinforce.

This is not to say that Egypt's resilient authoritarianism is on the verge of collapse, as it takes more that popular uprisings and international criticism to implement actual regime change. Nevertheless, what needs to be taken away when analyzing the impact of COVID-19 on Egyptian society and political institutions is that there are small, structural changes that have indeed begun to take place. The key role of civil society and institutions in developing strategies and policies to combat the epidemic signals a significant step back of the military forces and is a prime example of an internal shift of power within the country's political institutions. Meaningful social and political change takes time; however, the outbreak of the pandemic and its impact on state-society relations in Egypt might be signaling that this is indeed on the cards. Moving forward, it is crucial to keep an eye on how the regime's escalating authoritarianism is perceived regionally and internationally, to further investigate what forces might be working beneath the surface. The repercussions from the pandemic, an ongoing economic crisis and unrelenting demographic growth require concrete and quick answers from the regime. In this increasingly unstable context, any societal fracture exasperated by a brutal crackdown has the potential to deliver a significant blow to resilient authoritarianism.

Notes

1 Ketchley, N. (2017) *Egypt in a Time of Revolution* (Cambridge: Cambridge University Press); Wickham, C. (2013) *The Muslim Brotherhood: The Evolution of an Islamist Movement* (Princeton, NJ: Princeton University Press); Bassiouni, C. (2016) "Egypt's unfinished revolution", in A. Roberts, M. Willis, R. McCarthy, and T. Garton-Ash (eds.), *Civil Resistance in the Arab Spring: Triumphs and Disasters* (Oxford: Oxford University Press), pp. 53–88; Ottaway, M. (2003) *Democracy Challenged: The Rise of Semi-Authoritarianism* (Washington, DC: Carnegie Endowment for International Peace).

2 Pratt, N. and Rezk, D. (2019), "Securitizing the Muslim brotherhood: state violence and authoritarianism in Egypt after the Arab Spring", *Security Dialogue* 50:3, pp. 239–256.

3 Gramsci, A. (1971) *Selections from the Prison Notebooks*, Trans. and ed. by Hoare Q. and Nowell-Smith G. (London: Lawrence and Wishart), p. 258.

4 Pratt and Rezk, "Securitizing the Muslim Brotherhood".

5 Allman, K. (2018) "Revolution and counter-revolution in Egypt's emergency state", *OxHRH Blog*, http://ohrh.law.ox.ac.uk/revolution-and-counterrevolution-in-egypts- emergency-state/

6 Ardovini, L. and Mabon, S. (2020) "Egypt's unbreakable curse: tracing the State of Exception from Mubarak to Al Sisi", *Mediterranean Politics*, 25:4, p. 463.

7 Ibid., p. 466.

8 Stork, J. (2014) "Egypt: painting 'terrorism' with a very broad brush", *Human Rights Watch*, http://www.hrw.org/news/2014/05/05/egyptpainting-terrorism-very-broad-brush

9 Guerin, O. (2018) "The shadow over Egypt", *BBC News*, (23 February), https://www.bbc.co.uk/news/resources%20/idt-sh/shadow_over_egypt

10 Human Rights Watch (2020) "Egypt: COVID_19 cover for new repressive powers", https://www.hrw.org/news/2020/05/07/egypt-covid-19-cover-new-repressive-powers#

11 Euromed Rights (2020) "COVID-19: a new Trojan horse to step up authoritarianism in Egypt", https://euromedrights.org/publication/covid-19-a-new-trojan-horse-to-step-up-authoritarianism-in-egypt/

12 Albrecht, H. (2012), "Authoritarian transformation or transition from authoritarianism? Insights on regime change in Egypt", in Korany, B. and El-Mahdi, R. (eds.) *Arab Spring in Egypt: Revolution and Beyond* (Cairo: Cairo University Press), pp. 251–252.

13 Al Jazeera (2019) "In rare protests, Egyptians demand President el-Sisi's removal", (21 September) https://www.aljazeera.com/news/2019/09/21/in-rare-protests-egyptians-demand-president-el-sisis-removal/

14 World Health Organization, "COVID-19: Egypt" https://covid19.who.int/region/emro/country/eg

15 Mezran, K., Melcangi, A., Burchfield, E. and Riboua, Z. (2020) "The coronavirus crisis highlights the unique challenges of North African countries", *Atlantic Council*, (30 March) https://www.atlanticcouncil.org/blogs/mena-source/the-coronavirus-crisis-highlights-the-unique-challenges-of-north-african-countries/?fbclid=IwAR09DWItqDe_alCZDdtssp3i5ejZWVN4C-Qf45kn2Twj0r4V-Cp0Hz0kYBCA

16 Middle East Eye (2020) "Panic in Luxor: Coronavirus outbreak in Egypt found to be centred on ancient city", (11 March) https://www.middleeasteye.net/news/coronavirus-egypt-luxor-panic-epicentre-outbreak-tourism

17 Oztas, T. (2020) "Novel Coronavirus: stress test for Egypt's fragile economy", *AA*, (31 March), https://www.aa.com.tr/en/analysis/opinion-novel-coronavirus-stress-test-for-egypt-s-fragile-economy/1786298

18 Ardovini, L. (2020a) "COVID-19 in Egypt: global pandemics in times of authoritarianism", *ISPI*, (09 April) https://www.ispionline.it/en/pubblicazione/covid-19-egypt-global-pandemics-times-authoritarianism-25653

19 Al Arabiya (2020) "Egypt's mega-city Cairo shuts down for coronavirus curfew", (March 2020) https://english.alarabiya.net/en/News/middle-east/2020/03/26/Egypt-s-mega-city-Cairo-shuts-down-for-coronavirus-curfew-.html

20 Breisinger, C., Raouf, M., Wiebelt, M., Kamaly, A. and Karara, M. (2020) "Impact of COVID-19 on the Egyptian economy: economic sectors, jobs, and households", *IFPRI Middle East and North Africa*, pp. 1–12.

21 France 24 (2020), "Going viral: Arab world treats virus panic with humour", (12 March) https://www.france24.com/en/20200312-going-viral-arab-world-treats-virus-panic-with-humour

22 Ardovini, L. (2020b) "Resilient authoritarianism and global pandemics: challenges in Egypt at the time of COVID-19", *POMEPS: The COVID-19 Pandemics in North Africa and the Middle East*, https://pomeps.org/resilient-authoritarianism-and-global-pandemics-challenges-in-egypt-at-the-time-of-covid-19#_edn6

23 Amin, S. (2020) "Egypt battles COVID-19 amid flood of misinformation, conspiracy theories", *al Monitor*, (31 March) https://www.al-monitor.com/pulse/originals/2020/03/egyptian-superstitions-jokes-on-coronavirus.html#ixzz6IRcMSSUj

24 Ardovini, "Resilient authoritarianism and global pandemics".

25 Al Jazeera (2020) "Egypt arrests activists demanding prisoners are freed amid virus", (19 March) https://www.aljazeera.com/news/2020/03/19/egypt-arrests-activists-demanding-prisoners-are-freed-amid-virus/

26 Al Jazeera (2020) "Egypt targets Guardian, NYT journalists over coronavirus reports", (18 March) https://www.aljazeera.com/news/2020/03/18/egypt-targets-guardian-nyt-journalists-over-coronavirus-reports/?utm_source=website&utm_medium=article_page&utm_campaign=read_more_links; Michaelson, R., (2020a) "Egypt: rate of coronavirus cases 0likely to be higher than figures suggest'", *The Guardian*, (15 March) https://www.theguardian.com/world/2020/mar/15/egypt-rate-coronavirus-cases-higher-than-figures-suggest

27 Ardovini, "COVID-19 in Egypt".

28 Tran, E. (2020) "2020: the year of authoritarianism in the Middle East", *International Review*, https://international-review.org/2020-the-year-of-authoritarianism-the-middle-east/
29 Michaelson, R. (2020b) "Egypt cracking down harder on human rights groups, experts say", *The Guardian*, (23 November) https://www.theguardian.com/world/2020/nov/23/egypt-cracking-down-harder-on-human-rights-groups-experts-say
30 Joe Biden, Twitter (12 July 2020) https://twitter.com/joebiden/status/1282419453939113989?lang=en
31 Middle East Monitor (2020) "Egypt: opponents say Sisi's rule as dangerous as coronavirus", (23 March) https://www.middleeastmonitor.com/20200323-egypt-opponents-say-sisis-rule-as-dangerous-as-coronavirus/
32 Brown, N. and Hamzawy, A. (2020) "The role of Egypt's Armed Forces: a Military Empire", *ISPI*, p. 8.
33 Ibid.
34 Gervasio, G. and Teti, A., (2020) "Egypt's repression against civil society", *ISPI*, p. 17.

References

Al Arabiya (2020) "Egypt's mega-city Cairo shuts down for coronavirus curfew", (March 2020) https://english.alarabiya.net/en/News/middle-east/2020/03/26/Egypt-s-mega-city-Cairo-shuts-down-for-coronavirus-curfew-.html

Albrecht, H. (2012), "Authoritarian transformation or transition from authoritarianism? Insights on regime change in Egypt", in Korany, B. and El-Mahdi, R. (eds.) *Arab Spring in Egypt: Revolution and Beyond* (Cairo: Cairo University Press), pp. 251–252.

Al Jazeera (2019) "In rare protests, Egyptians demand President el-Sisi's removal", (21 September) https://www.aljazeera.com/news/2019/09/21/in-rare-protests-egyptians-demand-president-el-sisis-removal/

Al Jazeera (2020a) "Egypt arrests activists demanding prisoners are freed amid virus", (19 March) https://www.aljazeera.com/news/2020/03/19/egypt-arrests-activists-demanding-prisoners-are-freed-amid-virus/

Al Jazeera (2020b) "Egypt targets Guardian, NYT journalists over coronavirus reports" (18 March) https://www.aljazeera.com/news/2020/03/18/egypt-targets-guardian-nyt-journalists-over-coronavirus-reports/?utm_source=website&utm_medium=article_page&utm_campaign=read_more_links

Allman, K. (2018) "Revolution and counter-revolution in Egypt's emergency state", *OxHRH Blog*, http://ohrh.law.ox.ac.uk/revolution-and-counterrevolution-in-egypts- emergency-state/

Amin, S. (2020) "Egypt battles COVID-19 amid flood of misinformation, conspiracy theories", *al Monitor*, (31 March) https://www.al-monitor.com/pulse/originals/2020/03/egyptian-superstitions-jokes-on-coronavirus.html#ixzz6IRcMSSUj

Ardovini, L. (2020a) "COVID-19 in Egypt: global pandemics in times of authoritarianism", *ISPI*, (09 April) https://www.ispionline.it/en/pubblicazione/covid-19-egypt-global-pandemics-times-authoritarianism-25653

Ardovini, L. (2020b) "Resilient authoritarianism and global pandemics: challenges in Egypt at the time of COVID-19", *POMEPS: The COVID-19 Pandemics in North Africa and the Middle East*, https://pomeps.org/resilient-authoritarianism-and-global-pandemics-challenges-in-egypt-at-the-time-of-covid-19#_edn6

Ardovini, L. and Mabon, S. (2020) "Egypt's unbreakable curse: tracing the State of Exception from Mubarak to Al Sisi", *Mediterranean Politics*, 25:4, p. 463.

Bassiouni, C. (2016) "Egypt's unfinished revolution", in A. Roberts, M. Willis, R. McCarthy, and T. Garton-Ash (eds.), *Civil Resistance in the Arab Spring: Triumphs and Disasters* (Oxford: Oxford University Press).

Breisinger, C., Raouf, M., Wiebelt, M., Kamaly, A. and Karara, M. (2020) "Impact of COVID-19 on the Egyptian economy: economic sectors, jobs, and households", *IFPRI Middle East and North Africa*, Policy Note 6, pp. 1–12.

Brown, N. and Hamzawy, A. (2020) "The role of Egypt's Armed Forces: a Military Empire", *Italian Institute for International Political Studies (ISPI)*, Milan, Italy.

Euromed Rights (2020) "COVID-19: a new Trojan horse to step up authoritarianism in Egypt", https://euromedrights.org/publication/covid-19-a-new-trojan-horse-to-step-up-authoritarianism-in-egypt/

France 24 (2020) "Going viral: Arab world treats virus panic with humour", (12 March) https://www.france24.com/en/20200312-going-viral-arab-world-treats-virus-panic-with-humour

Gervasio, G. and Teti, A. (2020) "Egypt's repression against civil society", *ISPI*.

Gramsci, A. (1971) *Selections from the Prison Notebooks*, Trans. and ed. by Hoare Q. and Nowell-Smith G. (London: Lawrence and Wishart).

Guerin, O. (2018) "The shadow over Egypt", *BBC News*, (23 February) https://www.bbc.co.uk/news/resources%20/idt-sh/shadow_over_egypt

Human Rights Watch (2020) "Egypt: COVID_19 cover for new repressive powers", https://www.hrw.org/news/2020/05/07/egypt-covid-19-cover-new-repressive-powers#

Joe Biden, Twitter (12 July 2020) https://twitter.com/joebiden/status/1282419453939113989?lang=en

Ketchley, N. (2017) *Egypt in a Time of Revolution* (Cambridge: Cambridge University Press).

Mezran, K., Melcangi, A., Burchfield, E. and Riboua, Z. (2020) "The coronavirus crisis highlights the unique challenges of North African countries", *Atlantic Council*, (30 March) https://www.atlanticcouncil.org/blogs/menasource/the-coronavirus-crisis-highlights-the-unique-challenges-of-north-african-countries/?fbclid=IwAR09DWItqDe_alCZDdtssp3i5ejZWVN4CQf45kn2Twj0r4V-Cp0Hz0kYBCA

Michaelson, R. (2020a) "Egypt: rate of coronavirus cases likely to be higher than figures suggest", *The Guardian*, (15 March) https://www.theguardian.com/world/2020/mar/15/egypt-rate-coronavirus-cases-higher-than-figures-suggest

Michaelson, R. (2020b) "Egypt cracking down harder on human rights groups, experts say", *The Guardian*, (23 November) https://www.theguardian.com/world/2020/nov/23/egypt-cracking-down-harder-on-human-rights-groups-experts-say

Middle East Eye (2020) "Panic in Luxor: Coronavirus outbreak in Egypt found to be centred on ancient city", (11 March) https://www.middleeasteye.net/news/coronavirus-egypt-luxor-panic-epicentre-outbreak-tourism

Middle East Monitor (2020) "Egypt: opponents say Sisi's rule as dangerous as coronavirus", (23 March) https://www.middleeastmonitor.com/20200323-egypt-opponents-say-sisis-rule-as-dangerous-as-coronavirus/

Ottaway, M. (2003) *Democracy Challenged: The Rise of Semi-Authoritarianism* (Washington, DC: Carnegie Endowment for International Peace).

Oztas, T. (2020) "Novel Coronavirus: stress test for Egypt's fragile economy", *AA*, (31 March), https://www.aa.com.tr/en/analysis/opinion-novel-coronavirus-stress-test-for-egypt-s-fragile-economy/1786298

Pratt, N. and Rezk, D. (2019) "Securitizing the Muslim brotherhood: state violence and authoritarianism in Egypt after the Arab Spring", *Security Dialogue* 50:3, pp. 239–256.

Stork, J. (2014) "Egypt: Painting 'terrorism' with a very broad brush", *Human Rights Watch*, http://www.hrw.org/news/2014/05/05/egyptpainting-terrorism-very-broad-brush

Tran, E. (2020) "2020: the year of authoritarianism in the Middle East", *International Review*, https://international-review.org/2020-the-year-of-authoritarianism-the-middle-east/

Wickham, C. (2013) *The Muslim Brotherhood: The Evolution of an Islamist movement* (Princeton, NJ: Princeton University Press).

World Health Organization (2020) "COVID-19: Egypt" https://covid19.who.int/region/emro/country/eg

6 Iran's Bottom-Up Efforts and Challenges throughout the COVID-19 Pandemic

Ali Maleki and Najmoddin Yazdi

Introduction

Since late 2019, the world has been plagued by the COVID-19 pandemic. Because this crisis is essentially different from prior crises, it can serve as a good benchmark for the efficiency of governance institutions, governments' responses to the crisis, and crisis management. To begin, this crisis has occurred on a worldwide scale, and all countries have been complicit in it for an extended period of time, thereby eliminating the possibility of receiving assistance from other countries to overcome human, financial, and equipment resource constraints. Additionally, this characteristic enables countries' responses to the crisis to be substantially comparable. There is no such similarity in natural calamities such as hurricanes, sandstorms, volcanoes, earthquakes, and forest fires, in which towns and countries can rely on the assistance of other areas and countries. The second major difference is that it is a contagious situation, which severely restricts the action and presence of people and non-governmental forces due to the requirements for quarantine and physical distancing, as well as the complex dynamics of human mortality influenced by government policies. It is a dichotomous fight between economy and health, or in other words between food and life.

One of the primary issues in this sort of unusual crisis is acute resource scarcity, which cannot be resolved by infusing the limited resources of governments – regardless of their wealth – because society requires material and human resources much more than is achievable and of course promptly. On the other hand, while the historical tendency of governance modes is toward more distributive, horizontal, and flat structures, the experience of this pandemic suggests that these new governance modes – and even the meta-governance mode – are incapable of fully responding to such global catastrophes.

Iran's experience with the COVID-19 outbreak was different in some senses from that of other countries, which adds to the study's attractiveness, specifically, the critical role of ordinary people in resolving the situation.

DOI: 10.4324/9781003266259-6

While Iran has endured decades of unprecedented economic, political, commercial, and financial sanctions, the Islamic Republic of Iran is now in a precarious economic situation (high inflation, a large fiscal deficit, and negative economic growth), and its per capita medical staff and facilities (such as hospital beds) are significantly lower than those of many other countries (World Bank, 2017, 2018). Per capita resources are viewed as critical during times of crisis, when rivalry for physical, human, and financial resources rises on a worldwide scale. The question that arises is how, in the midst of the Corona crisis, Iran witnessed a massive presence of individuals making heroic sacrifices rather than insurgency or the collapse of the regime. What were the specific activities, features, and challenges of Iran's reaction to the COVID-19 crisis, which were based on community groups capable of mitigating crises and mobilizing societal resources?

To address this question, the current article provides a brief theoretical background on bottom-up responses to crises and an overview of the Iranian cultural environment, which drives such bottom-up, popular responses to crises. Following that, the activities of Iranian volunteer community groups are portrayed through seven axes, employing grounded theory and in-depth interviews with prominent players. Finally, the authors discuss the challenges that have surfaced in Iran's bottom-up response to crises.

Theoretical Background

In times of crisis, particularly large-scale or severe crises, citizens and thinkers are constantly focused on the efficacy and necessity of the government's extensive engagement in the crisis (Grube, 2020; Grube & Storr, 2014). However, it is commonly recognized that governments do not always perform as intended (Mises, 1990; Hayek, 1945) and that local organizations and grassroots groups should in many cases enter the fray. In fact, governments, like individuals and groups, face three challenges: access to field information and available resources, prioritization of actions, and adaptability to changing or previously inexperienced conditions. In these instances, popular groups can leverage their social capital, network, skills, and knowledge to collect field data more quickly and with greater quality from available challenges and resources while also coordinating with one another (Chamlee-Wright, 2010; Hurlbert et al., 2000; Storr et al., 2016). Three pillars support this direction: knowledge sharing, error correction, and social learning (Chamlee-Wright, 2010; Storr et al., 2016, 2017). And that the accumulation and repetition of these experiences throughout time results in the building of resilient societies (Aldrich, 2012; Burton, 2015; Chamlee-Wright, 2010).

Bottom-up recovery efforts involve putting various resources, such as goods, services, and information, in front of those in need, coordinating the process, and getting the community involved, since this approach can tap into local knowledge, harness and leverage social capital, and deal with rapidly changing circumstances (Grube, 2020). Although disaster assistance was traditionally handled at the community level until the early twentieth century, governments today recognize and promote public-private partnerships, business collaboration, and, on occasion, citizen engagement in disaster relief (Haeffele & Storr, 2020). The renewed focus on civil participation and collaborative public administration has made its way into the crisis management literature. In a broader context, public engagement has been a critical component of the conceptual shift in governance concepts, with deliberative and collective action techniques demonstrating the most promise (Cooper et al., 2006).

The term "citizen-driven reaction" has just recently begun to appear in the crisis management literature (e.g., see Bodin & Nohrstedt, 2016; Bodin et al., 2019; Correia et al., 2020; French, 2011; Goulding et al., 2018; Kapucu, 2015; Kapucu & Ustun, 2018; McLennan, 2020). The idea of faith-based civic participation, which this research highlighted as the bedrock of Iran's pandemic response, has gotten far less attention (the only instances the authors found, see Greyling et al., 2016; Rivera & Nickels, 2014). However, the results of Pratt et al. (2018) showed that when there is extreme uncertainty, fostering and sustaining leaps of faith is important for trust. Re-reading previous social capital and trust studies in crisis management and bottom-up response might therefore help understand the role of faith in civic involvement in emergencies, disasters, and crises.

Methods

The data gathering techniques used were semi-structured interviews, document analysis, and attendance at relevant webinars on Iran's bottom-up response to crises. In all, 26 interviews were conducted. The interviews, which lasted between 15 and 120 minutes apiece, were conducted over a four-month period. All interviewees consented to being recorded on audio. The 'raw data' was created by combining all notes and audio recordings.

Interviewees (see Table 6.1) served in a variety of capacities during the COVDI-19 crisis and, in the majority of cases, during previous natural disasters throughout the country, including practitioner, volunteer citizen, public administrator, NGO leader or manager, jihadi group activist, clergy, student volunteer, faculty member, or public policy expert. They were picked through snowball sampling until the data collection reached a theoretical saturation point. Throughout the epidemic and prior crises in Iran, more than half of them held senior public or civic administration roles at the national or provincial level.

Table 6.1 Interviewees

Interview no.	Age	Education	Position	Organization
1	43	Hawzah Master of Islam History	Chairman of Trustees	Imamzadeh mosque
2	23	Master student in Electrical Eng.	CEO	Charity
3	24	Bachelor of Electrical Eng.	Secretariat	Student Heyat
4	52	Master of Electrical Eng.	Founder; CEO	Medical device company
5	30	Diploma	CEO	Charity
6	32	MBA	CEO	Charity
7		Hawzah Bachelor	Manager	NGO
8	39	PhD of Political Science	Faculty member	Research institute
9	39	Doctor of Medicine	Faculty member	University
10	37	Master of Crisis Management	Instructor; Volunteer	Iranian Red Crescent
11	37	PhD of Technology Management	Founder; CEO	Medical device company
12	45	Hawzah Master of Religion	Public Manager	Provincial Hawzah
13	39	High School Diploma	Founder; CEO	Heyat
14	36	Master of Industrial Eng.	Manager	Jihadi group
15	36	MBA	Co-founder and CEO	Charity
16	35	Master	Founder and manager	High school
17	33	Master of Economics	Business consultant; Charity owner and manager	Charity; Jihadi group
18	50	High School Diploma	Founder	Home-made herbal medicine shop
19	45	Master	Co-founder	Heyat; Charity
20	35	Master of Industrial Eng.	Activist	-
21	30	Hawzah Bachelor	Clergy volunteer	Cemetery
22	40	PhD of Economics	Policy analyst	Think tank
23	37	Master of Industrial Eng.	Public servant	Public investment company
24	28	High School Diploma	Founder and CEO	Jihadi group
25	34	Master of Industrial Eng.	Executive officer	Private company
26	38	Master of Religion Studies	Manager	University student organization

Context: Religious Faith, Altruism and Trust

The Culture of Help (Farhang-e Yarigari in Persian) and the backdrop of altruism in Iranian civilization date all the way back several millennia (Interview 8; See also Farhadi, 2002), which has been resurrected in recent decades through the concepts of 'jihadi management' and 'jihadi approach' (for a recent work, see Hasani Nik & Mokhtarianpour, 2019). Despite the increase in individuality brought about by modernity's advent in Iran during the last half-century, this culture has not only remained intact but has also reached its zenith during the Islamic Revolution (1978) and Iraq's eight-year war inflicted on Iran (the Holy Defense). During the Holy Defense, enormous numbers of volunteers from across the country journeyed to the south and west to defend the borders; women and the elderly, who were unable to join the warriors on the front, assisted the soldiers by sending food, clothing, and other supplies.

Following the war, the country has had the experiences of Construction Jihad, popular Basij bases, and the involvement of popular and jihadi groups in the management of natural catastrophes such as floods, earthquakes, and hurricanes, all of which continue to operate in normal times as well as during times of crisis. Numerous countries have witnessed the presence of voluntary grassroots groups during times of crisis. However, this approach is peculiar for Iran, as studies occasionally reflect a decline in public trust and social capital in the country, which has been eroding for the last 2–3 decades. According to surveys, the Iranian people feel gloomy about themselves and the government (for example, see Gallup World Poll, 2020). Zucker (1986) defined trust broadly as "a set of expectations shared by all those involved in the exchange." Yamagishi and Yamagishi (1994) called trust "a belief in the benevolence of human nature in general."

Experts usually agree that trust is a necessary component of cooperative conduct. On the other hand, there is a substantial body of studies demonstrating how involvement in social life results in improved trust (Paxton & Ressler, 2018). Thus, a paradox arises regarding how people contribute in times of crisis (and even in normal circumstances) despite their pessimism and distrust. There are two possible explanations. One is that without trust, cooperation and participation of the populace are possible in times of acute peril or collective terror. The second interpretation is that this participation would not have occurred in the absence of trust, but the definition of trust should be expanded to encompass not only rational trust but also faith-based trust (including religious faith). When people are present in non-crisis situations, the second explanation appears to be more sensible. Indeed, people's response to catastrophes, such as the COVID-19 pandemic, is primarily motivated by a sense of spiritual and religious duty, rather than rational calculation, livelihood wisdom, or civic responsibility as a modern notion. In the perspective of the majority of the public, the government is legitimate and trustworthy despite its flaws and dysfunctions.

It has been consistently demonstrated in classical research that faith communities have significantly greater social capital as a result of their shared rituals, essence, stories, experiences, risks, or understandings (Pratt et al., 2018). Recently, faith has been defined as a component of trust building (such as Pratt et al., 2018). These studies, however, do not always define it as religious faith; they may also encompass instinctive feelings of nationalism, sacrifice, and humanity. Field observations in Iran suggest that religious faith is used to shape trust and social capital, which are inherently more prevalent among religious and jihadi organizations such as mosque-based communities and Heyats. It is possible to hypothesize that in Iranian society, non-religious faith is more effective in bringing that segment of the population to the point of expressing disgust and opposition to events or decisions that are unfavorable to them than taking a constructive approach and assisting others in solving problems and dealing with crises.

The aforementioned paradox is raised again when discussing public trust in the government: how people have a strong belief in the government's inefficiency and the bureaucratic system of Iran, but simultaneously defend its legitimacy and, in times of crisis, are not only indebted to the government but also willing to cooperate and assist it as much as possible voluntarily. The natural response is that religious faith instills trust in the legitimacy and health of the state, but not in its effectiveness. Indeed, the interviewees consistently reported that the government does not interfere adequately and should play a more supportive role, which indicates popular trust and acceptance of the government's function while believing in the inefficiencies of its structures, procedures, and servants.

To these complications must be added the decades-long economic, defense, and even pharmaceutical restrictions imposed by the United States, which contributed to the country's catastrophic economic situation throughout the pandemic. It resulted in currency devaluations, extraordinary unemployment rates, a lack of access to a number of critical medicines, and a prohibition on any money transfers, even humanitarian ones. Each of the aforementioned factors appears to be adequate to explain not only a country's citizens' non-participation – particularly during times of crisis – but also popular unrest and the demise of regime. Nonetheless, we continue to see the selfless and volunteer acts of popular groups, including those willing to visit hospitals, residences, and nursing homes where COVID-19 patients are treated or dwell, as well as the Islamic burial of deceased patients (including washing, shrouding, etc.).

Popular Activities

Civic groups' activity during the pandemic can be classified into seven categories: (1) Financing, purchasing, and distributing foodstuffs; (2) Health measures, including public disinfection and cleaning; (3) Organizing

ceremonies and gatherings in accordance with COVID-19 observations;
(4) Assisting health staff in hospitals and other settings; (5) Providing specialized or knowledge-based services and products; (6) Cultural, promotional, and educational measures; and (7) Empowerment of the vulnerable,
popular actors, and decision makers. The next sections provide evidence
and examples of interviews for each of these dimensions.

Financing, Purchasing, and Distributing Foodstuffs

From the start of the crisis, religious Heyats, popular groups, charities, and
non-governmental organizations (NGOs) began receiving popular money
by publicizing (mainly confirmed) bank account numbers. Provision of food
to vulnerable and impoverished families around the country is one of the
first and most prevalent initiatives taken by these actors in response to every
crisis. Popular groups are able to raise finances and assistance through their
networks of friends, neighbors, relatives, and other community members
who trust or are connected with them. They begin purchasing foodstuffs
in bulk in order to take advantage of considerable discounts – up to 50% –
offered by factories, major chain stores, and wholesalers. Occasionally,
these suppliers contribute additional savings to these charity efforts. These
are then delivered freely to disadvantaged families and crisis victims. Typically, this popular response lasts between one and three months following
natural disasters, but in a crisis such as the pandemic, it has been repeated
and has lasted so far, i.e., for more than a year. The majority of these groups
provide this service throughout the year, albeit on a more restricted basis.

According to the CEO of one of the charities, despite the fact that many
people were unemployed or in severe economic situations, financial aid
to our organization increased tenfold, owing in large part to the Supreme
Leader's call for Faithful Aid Movement. This resulted in a 12-fold increase
in food distribution. As a result, we required a rapid increase in the number
of our volunteer staff on the one hand (the supply side) and a rapid expansion of the target community on the other (the demand side) within a few
days, which we accomplished by quickly forming new collaborations with
other jihadi groups and charities (Interview 5). Interviewee 6 related the
same story. As the director of a youth charity in the capital, he claimed that
for the first time during the Corona crisis, we gave health kits containing
face masks, disinfectants, and detergents in addition to the customary food
packages. This was around 1,000 packets during the 2020 Ramadan month
and 600 packs during the Eid al-Ghadir festival, i.e., six to ten times the
normal activity (Interview 6).

The manager of a mosque-based, university-based, middle-sized civic
population in Tehran revealed that during the holy month of Ramadan
alone, we distributed over 10,000 packs in 14 provinces, which was accomplished with the assistance of 150–200 volunteers. They were willing to
spend the Iranian New Year apart from their family, putting themselves at

risk for getting a new sickness (Interview 3). In Yazd, clerics were able to fund and deliver over 10,000 food parcels thanks to the critical function of the mosque network (Interview 12).

For the composition of the food parcels, two shifts were detected. First, some popular groups, in accordance with the National Health Headquarters' Corona Protocols, began serving only cold and dry foodstuffs (Interviews 1 and 12), while others, such as university-based groups, questioned the reasoning (Interviews 3) or did not respond to it silently (Interview 13). They sought to give hot meals and fresh meat to the vulnerable as a necessity. Naturally, preparing and distributing hot meals and fresh meat has a considerable perceived benefit in society and among the poor. Second, in recent years, the variety of food packages has gradually increased, moving away from stereotypical products such as rice, oil, and sugar toward also tomato paste, meat, legumes, dates, and other goods. The groups, which were mostly made up of undergraduate and graduate volunteers, were said to have an interactive contact with the vulnerable families, allowing them to update and customize the needs and packages on a monthly basis. Stationery, clothing, and health kits are all examples of items that may be included in the shipments. These groups are primarily family-focused, with the goal of covering as many of their needs as possible in a comprehensive and dynamic manner (Interview 25).

Despite the intensification of financial pressures and unemployment, family-oriented groups that had joined the field of organic food and healthy eating before to the Corona crisis continued to give services to their covered family network. They increased their delivery of hot meals and fresh meat during religious holidays such as Ramadan, Eid Ghadir (Alavi feeding), and Eid al-Adha (Ikram Razavi). Cost savings in meat preparation are typically realized by these groups slaughtering sheep and calves themselves while adhering to sanitary standards (Interview 13).

To quickly and widely but reliably identify new needy people who have become vulnerable to the pandemic, jihadi groups ask assistance from other distribution and charitable networks, often with a representative of the financier or supplier present during the distribution process to the newly introduced unknown networks. Distribution through hospitals' Help Desks and school administrators are two more reliable strategies that ensure accurate information about the target groups (Interview 15).

Public Health Measures

Popular groups and individuals began disinfecting streets and public spaces such as mosques, shrines, and schools. They encountered ambiguities and complications as a result of their lack of prior experience, training, and necessary equipment. Interviewee 6 stated that we used to disinfect poverty stricken or crowded urban areas from night to morning using specific clothing and equipment. This continued for approximately three months until doubts about its effectiveness and priority were raised, at which point it was dropped from our and many other groups' priorities. A cleric in charge of an Imamzadeh (i.e., a sacred shrine) in one of Tehran's villages reported that volunteer jihadi groups came every other day to cleanse the Imamzadeh so that it could continue to serve the surrounding community and travelers. Furthermore, the provision of face masks and disposable gloves, as well as the placement of pedal disinfecting liquid at the shrine's entry, as well as the physical separation of the clients, allowed the shrine to continue its operations. This was one of the villagers' concerns (Interview 1). Certain traditional or religious organizations were averse to modern chemical disinfection methods and hence depended on traditional treatments, such as disinfecting surfaces with a mixture of vinegar, salt, and rose water rather than alcohol (Interview 7). At the local level, mosques and community mobilizations were active networks in distributing face masks and disinfection solutions. According to Interviewee 14:

> Our local mosque acquired raw materials for making face masks from the Execution of Imam Khomeini's Order (EIKO) and delivered to local housewives who volunteered to create face masks at home with their sewing machines. During the Iranian New Year vacations, one of the local tailors temporarily donated his workshop to the mosque, allowing ladies who do not own a sewing machine to make masks. I looked after our children for a several months so that my wife could attend the sewing workshop and assist with the sewing.

He adds that the Islamic Revolutionary Guard Corps (IRGC) and Basij's buying and distribution network aided us significantly in lowering prices, speeding up production, and minimizing trial and error. The director of a five-year-old charity noted:

> Supplying medicines to needy COVID-19 patients, providing ventilators to needy patients at home, and donating ventilators to hospitals were among our new activities during the pandemic's initial weeks.

He underlined that we did not go to offer face masks, protective clothing, or juice for the medical staff because we observed that other groups were meeting these necessities, and hence we went to the neglected needs.

Organizing Ceremonies and Gatherings

Religious rites, gatherings, and pilgrimages are vital to Iran's society, and as such, one of the primary worries since the outbreak has been how to keep these meetings going. From weekly home gatherings within the family network to regional and national religious gatherings and rituals at mosques, Hussainiyas, and Heyats, these events have become an integral part of

Iranian social life. These have undeniable theological, psychological, uniting, and epistemological value across the board – most notably among jihadi and civic groups engaged in crises, charities, and humanitarian efforts.

The efforts and innovations made by the public to keep these events going can be divided into three time periods. Initially, when nothing was known about the new virus and most people were concerned, the events were canceled in a conservative approach in accordance with the rules announced by the Ministry of Health. Meanwhile, many civic organizations have shifted their activities to internet platforms, including religious lectures, book readings, Quran recitations, mourning, and occasional celebrations (Interviews 1 and 3). Volunteer clerics began offering community members with telephone services on pandemic rulings and suspicions, as well as psychological counseling and reassurance, as well as visiting martyrs' families, the elderly, and medical personnel (Interview 12).

After a period of closure of religious sites and gatherings, demand for their reopening gradually increased in the second phase, and finally, with the support of the Supreme Leader, religious groups and citizens reopened the mosques, Heyats, and gatherings in accordance with the protocols issued by the Ministry of Health. Interestingly, protocol compliance was often higher in these locations than in other social settings such as public service offices, retail malls, bazaars, and public thoroughfares. Among the tactics implemented in the second phase were rituals with social distancing in open spaces, vast areas, or sometimes movable by vehicle in streets and alleyways (Interview 3). As an illustration, a religious charity organized a carnival for the youngsters of a peri-urban region of the capital that is densely populated with old brick kilns (Interview 24). Brick kilns, or facilities for manufacturing burnt clay bricks for construction, are common in Asia's peri-urban areas, including Iran. Such locations are frequently overly dirty, destitute, and the children are frequently forced to work in hazardous settings, such as brick kilns. Another organized a children's kite festival in Taft, a town located outside the capital (Interview 13).

However, in the third phase, some popular groups, particularly those with educated members, began to move ahead of protocols by scrutinizing them critically, serving as role models for other organizations, or even pushing provincial and national authorities to reform unnecessary and unproductive procedures (Interview 3). Family-oriented groups with no financial or institutional ties to (quasi-)governmental agencies sometimes adopted this third-phase strategy from the onset and never ceased their gatherings. Surprisingly, they self-reported having nil infection rates to us (Interview 13).

Assisting Health Staff

The popular backing of the medical staff was one of the most startling instances during the Corona crisis in Iran. This assistance was not simply a matter of verbal gratitude or media discourse. In a circumstance where many people remained in their houses, some self-sacrificing volunteers raced to their practical aid, even in the absence of suitable clothing and protective equipment. The spark for this creative effort comes from the Supreme Leader's support and description of medical personnel as 'defenders of health.' To appreciate the metaphor's cultural relevance, one must first grasp its history: Four decades ago, the martyrs and volunteers of Iraq's eight-year imposed war on Iran were dubbed 'defenders of the border' ('Harim' in Persian; i.e., the country). Then, during the last decade, in defense of the holy shrines and people of friendly neighboring countries such as Syria, Lebanon, Iraq, Yemen, and Palestine against terrorist groups or foreign enemies, the metaphor of 'defenders of the shrine' was used. The new metaphor of 'defenders of health' expands on the previous two metaphors by portraying the pandemic as a war, highlighting the importance of medical personnel's sacrifices and those who help them. This relation between four decades of self-sacrifice was confirmed by a war veteran who is now the CEO of a ventilator manufacturer (Interview 4). Another step in connecting these three analogies was the development of a photo show during Holy Defense Week with the slogan 'from yesterday to today' (Interview 12).

Many clergy volunteered at hospitals to provide relief, consolation, and psychological counseling to COVID-19 patients, as well as to teach religious rulings if necessary. In Yazd province alone, one of Iran's 31 provinces, 25 clerics rushed to assist hospital workers, and around 1,000 hours of counseling were performed (Interview 12). To the amazement of the Minister of Health, a number of volunteer clergy came to assist hospital workers, even providing cleaning and disinfection services (Interview 12). During the first 2–3 months of the crisis, various jihadi groups and charities routinely prepared and distributed daily hot meals, fruit juices, and snacks. As a result, parallel distribution and extra food and juice were occasionally noticed (Interviews 3 and 14). In addition, due to a shortage of alcohol, disinfectants, shields, and clothing, several groups volunteered to donate these supplies to hospitals' staff, particularly in the early months (Interviews 3 and 12).

Specialized or Knowledge-Based Services and Products

Along with social innovations, one of the most significant opportunities presented by the pandemic to the popular movement was the development of novel specialized, technical, engineering services and goods. For the first time, technological businesses came in to assist with crisis management, and this entry was, of course, beyond the simple logic of market profitability and cost-benefit analysis. For example, a medical equipment company, that took three years prior to the crisis to achieve European standards in the manufacture of simple ventilators through technology transfer, was able to rapidly and independently develop volume-synchronized intermittent mandatory ventilators (SIMV), a technology that is monopolized by a few advanced countries. Scaling up the production is more difficult than it appears.

For instance, new device testing typically takes 24 months (Penarredonda, 2020). However, the company pioneered rapid design of numerous components and increased total output by more than 30 times in less than three months for the first time (Interview 4):

> Developing and manufacturing an advanced ventilator for the first time without the assistance of technology companies is extremely complex and sensitive, as the final tests must be conducted clinically on a patient whose life is dependent on the device's operation. It was difficult to ask production, R&D, and after-sales staff to stay overnight at the company. Many of them should have gone to hospitals for testing and feedback, but they all agreed that we should do this jihad in the end. To fully utilize the company's capacity, we worked three shifts and tested and calibrated the parts at night. Among them were people who lived with pregnant spouses, infants, or elderly parents, putting their own lives at risk as well as their own. Prior to the Corona, the survival rate under our ventilators was 30%; During the Corona's early years (due to its unknown status and, of course, a lack of advanced technology), it dropped to 10%; But it has now increased to 50%. Our production machine costs one-fifth as much as the Chinese model. However, even if we had paid, no country would have given Iran a ventilator during the first few months because everyone needed it. Even during normal times, the US-led medical embargo on Iran posed an additional barrier to obtaining a ventilator.

According to Interviewee 11:

> The Pandemic was an opportunity to get involved in the maintenance of Computed Tomography (CT) scanners and ventilators that were desperately needed by COVID-19 patients, and was, of course, sanctioned. In fact, the crisis created a window of opportunity for policy change and demand; Previously, hospitals and the Ministry of Health were primarily looking to buy from abroad and, to a lesser extent, from within, with no serious demand for the maintenance and optimal use of existing devices. We discovered that we have over 2,700 ventilators stored in hospital warehouses, approximately 900 of which are repairable and returnable. The issue with CT scanners was a ban on spare parts, particularly consumable items and high-tech parts. For the first time in Iran, we assembled about 30 technical teams of the best experienced engineers and repairmen in less than a month to tackle a maintenance task that had been decided to ignore for the previous two decades.

According to him, the country is not confronted with insurmountable obstacles in terms of medical services and equipment supply. The challenge is with the demand side, where government agencies don't trust domestic capabilities and instead rely on foreign purchases as well as on long and inefficient license-issuing processes. The pandemic provided the government with an opportunity to demonstrate that licenses that had previously taken 2–3 years to issue could now be issued in as little as 1–6 months, and that domestic producers, entrepreneurs, and innovators could be trusted (Interview 11).

Another issue was the absence of a comprehensive and current database of vulnerable individuals. After years of government and quasi-government failure to create a comprehensive and up-to-date database of the needy, popular and governmental actors have found a long-established information technology (IT) company willing to offer a platform for the database. Meanwhile, one of the jihadi groups has created a limited but high-quality and reliable database that has become a reference point for other popular groups. Government databases, despite their extensive coverage, lack the necessary quality and up-to-datedness and are practically useless (Interview 5).

In another experiment, a university professor and co-founder of a technology company recounted his experience developing the nanofiber substrate for face masks and then building the country's first face mask production machine. He described his experience recruiting volunteers at the workshop production line during the pandemic's first six months (Interview 9):

> I approached my students, and ten volunteer medical students expressed interest in assisting us. On the other hand, the same number of priests from one of the seminaries (dubbed Hawzah) came to our help, quarantining themselves in the workshop for months. These people were always on a fast. The cultural divides between clergy and students were evident and concerning. However, by the end of the collaboration, the two groups were pleasantly surprised to discover that they understood each other much better. Despite the fact that my wife was pregnant and had a small child, I used to spend time with the volunteers, traveling 6–7 hours a day to and from the workshop outside of town, and returning home late at night when my family was sleeping. In those days, my family faced a significant risk of contracting the COVID-19 disease.

Cultural, Promotional, and Educational Measures

Popular groups' cultural, promotional, and educational efforts can be classified into four categories:

First, actions aimed at youth and students, such as providing stationery, providing tablets for students' virtual education, and instructing them (Interview 5);

Second, informing and raising awareness through cyberspace and media, as well as through multimedia works (Interview 12);

Third, individual or family-level competitions, festivals, and cultural, educational, or recreational competitions. These included puppet shows, the launch of mental and physical health promotion channels on social media, and the preparation and installation of banners, posters, and photographs for relaxing and educational purposes in passageways, bakeries, and bus stations. Among the other initiatives were the launch of 'Joy of Game' virtual channels for indoor family games, Quranic and prayer competitions, live Quran recitation on Instagram, Islamic counseling virtual channels, memoir contests, and the production of short promotional or educational TV programs and videoclips. There were numerous pre-prayer health training courses, ethics sessions, epistemological empowerment classes, and tailoring, embroidery, photography, photo editing, and video editing training classes for girls and women in the country-wide network of mosques (Interviews 1, 3, 12, and 13);

And fourth, when providing assistance, a special emphasis was placed on the self-esteem and dignity of those receiving assistance. One expression of this issue has been the omission of the charity's or civic group's logo and name from the meals supplied. At times, food packs were distributed in the bags of chain stores to protect needy individuals' reputation. However, governmental organizations refused to distribute their stuff without their trademark or logo (Interviews 2 and 6).

Empowerment of the Vulnerable, Popular Actors, and Decision Makers

Over the last decade, many Iranian jihadi actors have debated whether this kind of emergency resource use is sustainable or whether we should progressively transition toward more empowering and capability-building services. Furthermore, how? In this sense, there has been a trend among popular groups to lend Qard-al-Hasan loans to the needy rather than relying on grants all of the time. This was also true in the face of pandemic unemployment, when a variety of groups attempted to supply labor tools or raw materials to unemployed individuals (Interviews 5, 6, and 13). (For further study of the Iranian case of bottom-up Islamic social finance, see Yazdi et al., 2021.) In another move, several technological enterprises began manufacturing industrial face mask-making machinery for the first time, after recognizing that the jihadi groups' manual efforts were unable to satisfy the needs of society (Interview 9).

Traditional medicine groups also began freely providing free education and supporting the home manufacture of traditional and religious medicines, rather than simply attempting to create on their own and generate money through sales (Interviews 7 and 18). The aforementioned set of measures aimed to empower vulnerable populations, but some civic groups, particularly those with a university background, were more concerned with expanding their expertise and passing on their experiences to younger colleagues. This is empowerment of popular actors as opposed to empowerment of vulnerable target groups, which has been described previously. In these groups, when membership dynamics are significant, the transfer of experience and tacit knowledge is critical (Interviews 3 and 7). In addition, groups having a student body scrutinized practices and regulations. They used the informal channels at their disposal to offer ideas for policy and structure reform and change to national, provincial, and urban decision makers on a regular basis. Interestingly, public decision makers have occasionally turned to these groups to better grasp field realities and get local knowledge of policy implementation and implications (Interview 3).

Challenges

The popular response to Iran's COVID-19 issue demonstrated that bottom-up models may give rapid, flexible, unified, integrated, and comprehensive responses (i.e., encompassing a varied range of functions) that are based on field data (i.e., to have continuous feedback loops from the implementation level). These responses are founded on enablers such as popular leadership, popular actors' internal incentive systems, preserving the dignity of the needy and vulnerable, learning by doing, and empowering both actors and vulnerable (Marvi et al., 2021). However, Iran's experience suggests that this approach has major challenges to implementation and quality, which will be discussed below.

Lack of Information

One of the primary issues confronting grassroots and community groups in Iran is a lack of comprehensive and reliable data for identifying disadvantaged families and individuals (Interviews 5 and 25). While responsible government authorities have taken action in recent years, most interviewees stressed that this information is out of date and frequently inaccurate (e.g., Interview 5). Additionally, no information on the support received by each family is available, and the risk of a family receiving several contributions through different parallel channels is substantial. Popular groups mitigate this risk through their extensive local search, collaboration networks, and information sharing. To assist the truly needy, many of these groups rely on trusted local liaisons in each region to serve as their information backbone, thereby establishing a trustworthy, efficient information structure. Naturally, during times of crisis, popular groups must rely on completely new networks and information held by other jihadi groups, as the scope of their services must expand rapidly, the target community may be entirely new (as in the case of floods, earthquakes, and natural disasters that may occur elsewhere in the country), or new services must be offered that they have not previously offered.

Our colleagues in the Basij organization and the Islamic Revolutionary Guard Corps (IRGC) had vital information on the facilities, networks, groups, and distribution routes to share with us and a few other popular groups, according to Interviewee 14. The majority, however, did not have access to this information. Additionally, Interviewee 17 underlined the government's poor reporting on a range of problems, including safety guidelines for crisis management – particularly during natural disasters – and supporting victims. According to Interviewee 3, there is no platform established by government entities for getting field information from us, the crisis activists. Another significant concern has been civic groups' lack of participation in public decision-making and crisis management (Interview 3). Nonetheless, the society has seen the emergence of several bottom-up schemes to compensate for the government institutions' inadequacy in this area. For instance, the Hosseini Initiation Plan ('Ruyesh-e-Hosseini,' in Persian) enquires about people's concerns and then refers them to government authorities or those with the potential to address them (Interview 3). Another example is the bottom-up drafting of local development plans for neighborhoods based on their indigenous needs. In this end, with the support of the Imam Hussein University, a jihadi group active in Tehran's disadvantaged Darvaazeh Qaar neighborhood – which literally means Cave Gate – has prepared a local development plan (Interview 24). Finally, there is a dearth of knowledge about many vulnerable families who do not seek assistance due to their temperament. According to Interviewee 25, "You must come up with a solution to this problem. Perhaps the solution is to acquire and share information about such deserving families horizontally and from the bottom up."

Coordination and Cooperation Failure

Iran's public response to crises is characterized by a huge number of volunteers, various civic organizations, and a big number of charities. Interference and incoherence between these popular groups and the government, on the other hand, is one of the scourges plaguing Iran's bottom-up crisis responses. "In truth, we are currently in full chaos and require a great deal of centralization, orderliness, and coordination" (Interview 6). Coordination between civic groups and organizations is required to determine which tasks are necessary for which areas and how they are dispersed among the groups (Interview 6). For instance, parallel work is evident in the Mostazafan Foundation of Islamic Revolution, the Imam Khomeini Relief Foundation, and the Executive Headquarters of the Imam's Command – three organizations with significant resources and budgets for crisis management and assistance to the injured (Interviews 5 and 6). As another example, the government established the Heyat Online Platform to let civic groups conduct religious rites virtually during the pandemic, while the Islamic

Development Organization established the Tekyeh Online website concurrently. This was an example of public resources being wasted and parallel activities occurring throughout the pandemic (Interview 3).

A common fundamental issue is a lack of cooperation and contact between popular groups. However, coordination and cooperation between groups having young managers has improved significantly and has progressed, indicating a positive trend in this area (Interviews 10 and 15). Another issue is the lack of national goal-setting by government institutions, as well as supervision of the quality of services and goods offered by popular groups (Interview 14). Interviewee 24 pointed out that in communities where there are far more civic groups than are required, the diversity of actors has adverse implications. "Several entities were interfering with our production process independently and in parallel, including by seizing products and materials," Interviewee 9 said of his experience building a mask-making machine.

Government Dysfunctionality

One of the frequent themes of the interviews was people complaining about government institutions. For instance, Interviewee 1 indicated that "we did not receive assistance from official institutions in our immediate vicinity, such as this district's municipality, but jihadi groups from other locations came to our aid." Their priority is to take photos, report, and show off their achievements rather than to accomplish the task remaining on the ground; for this reason, we utterly abandoned them (Interview 1; also Interview 13). Government institutions have demonstrated that they lack both a strategy and compassion (Interview 16). In the field of education, Interviewee 16 stated the following:

> The quality of service provided by Shad Network – the exclusive school virtual education network – was so poor that individuals and schools switched to other domestic and international platforms; As a result, economies of scale were not achieved and inconsistencies intensified; Later, the Ministry of Education attempted to rectify this dysfunction by requiring schools to use Shad Network compulsorily.

According to Interviewee 10, an experienced aid worker with over ten years of teaching experience at one of the country's primary crisis management organizations:

> my organization, which is quasi-governmental rather than entirely popular, has a number of advantages, including strong international ties, a hierarchical structure, professional job descriptions, a sizable budget, and adequate facilities. However, varied behaviors and conversation are observed: during the pandemic, the primary topic of conversation among our colleagues was the points, degrees, and salaries that could be earned as a result of our activities, whether we would be promoted to

permanent employment, complaining about the mission's non-payment, and complaining about a lack of equipment and face masks. Due to the organization's continual competition with other crisis organizations, spectacular activities and a significant emphasis on media coverage of any action, no matter how minor, are priorities. In contrast with jihadi and civic groups which are often small and not officially registered, this dysfunction and malady exist in a large number of legally registered NGOs whose primary priority is media coverage and branding rather than crisis management or assisting the needy.

Interviewee 10 further explained:

> They approach crisis management from a political standpoint, to the extent where government agencies regard popular forces as adversaries and annoyances. This demonstrates the relevance of non-bureaucratic and non-governmental structures in strengthening popular and civic organisations.

In the early months, the Ministry of Health tended to cancel religious gatherings only one or two days before they were scheduled, despite having granted authorization to hold them. For religious groups and Heyats, it was extremely inconvenient and a waste of resources and energy; governments were supposed to make a single, earlier judgment in such circumstances (Interview 3). Furthermore, the Ministry of Health pursued its role in the pandemic regulation by mindlessly embracing global procedures rather than understanding and resolving it in detail based on local needs (Interview 3).

During this crisis, it became evident how complicated and difficult it is for technology to permeate our government structure, which serves as the primary purchaser of technological goods in times of crisis (Interview 23). One of the roadblocks in this regard is the requirement to get time-consuming permits in order to develop innovative goods and services (Interviews 11 and 23). Lack of support and even hindrance by governmental and quasi-governmental entities in the path of popular movements was frequently encountered; "We are pleased that government agencies do not simply walk into our shoes and leave us alone" (Interviews 7 and 9).

Interviewee 9 explained:

> The raw materials for our mask production were confiscated at customs, our workshop was repeatedly cut off, and the Basij forces confiscated our raw materials several times for hoarding; Meanwhile, the judiciary insisted on ordering us to work in three time shifts day and night while announcing any assistance to us. In comparison to my many years of volunteer experience in Canada, I have discovered that popular work in times of crisis in Iran truly takes iron shoes in terms of a lack of government services and support and a lack of a clearly defined role for popular forces.

Specialization and Learning

Previous crises were mostly natural calamities, and popular organizations brought their non-technological and non-specialty services, as well as their financial, human, and logistical resources, to the table. According to Interviewee 6:

> Specialized learning from previous experiences was always weak; currently, rather than their knowledge, specialty, or skills, it is the abundance and quantity of popular groups that solve the crisis; for times when the crisis becomes complex, we do not know what to do; in many crises, the groups have enough energy, but they do not know what exactly to do.

The lack of training courses and skills for crisis activists and popular groups was mentioned by Interviewee 17. Similarly, Interviewee 9 observed a lack of professional, consistent, and practical training to deal with the situation – particularly in light of his extensive volunteer experience in Canada. In this regard, Interviewee 14 offered the following example:

> Lack of training for home and novice forces in the early work of mask sewing workshops resulted in fabric waste and a significant learning period. Additionally, a lack of knowledge about the cost-benefit analysis of purchasing mask production equipment resulted in certain acquisitions that were not cost effective and ultimately ineffective. In certain circumstances, hand producing the masks proved more cost-effective than purchasing mask production machinery.

Specialized and technological responding to the crisis called for manufacturers to be able to obtain the raw materials and components they need in their production line in a short amount of time with the support of other manufacturers. In the production of ventilators, we had some cases of successful and quick collaboration with government organizations and companies (for example, in the innovative local battery supply), some cases of successful but too lengthy collaborations, and some cases of unsuccessful collaborations, according to Interviewee 4.

The COVID-19 pandemic provided Iran with an unprecedented chance to engage in the technological components of crisis response, in which technological businesses also play a role. Nonetheless, Interviewees 11 and 23 stressed the government agencies' and enterprises' reliance on overseas acquisitions and their lack of confidence in purchasing from domestic suppliers as a weakness of the demand side for technological goods. Crises, they argue, might provide as a window of opportunity to break this path dependency.

Empowerment: Root Response to Needs

The superficiality of popular groups and charities' solutions to the poor can be studied from both supply and demand perspectives. On the demand side, it is possible to detect a cultural poverty in which impoverished households disregard their spiritual, educational, and immaterial demands. For instance, according to Interviewee 25, a family may request funds to replace a burnt corner in a carpet or to purchase fashionable clothing and utensils, but healthy eating, kid education, and cultural expenses are not a priority. Correcting these views is a work that popular groups, as well as the media and public institutions, must undertake.

On the supply side, one of the issues is that groups have grown accustomed to providing monetary aid and food to the vulnerable rather than providing them with sustainable employment. Of course, this has shifted the preferences of recipients of aid and services in a cycle, to the point where they are more interested in receiving cash assistance and products than in being empowered and standing on their own two feet (Interview 3). Diversifying and tailoring services and goods to the specific needs of each family can serve as a first step in this direction (Interview 23). Three approaches – neighborhood-centered, family-centered, and comprehensive – can be integrated to create a root response. Civic organizations with roots in an area, as opposed to outside organizations that enter a neighborhood, offer more sustainable solutions with less negative consequences (Interview 24).

Conclusion

During the crisis, when the general public throughout the world, including Iran, and even some medical personnel, prioritized their own health and quarantined themselves at home or severely restricted their social activities, jihadi (popular) groups rushed to assist nurses, doctors, patients, needy families, and deceased bodies in hospitals, cemeteries, mosques, and charities. Indeed, for a long time, Iran's exposure to natural crises and emergency conditions has taken a different shape than traditional crisis responses – particularly in the four decades since the Islamic Revolution in the 1970s – so that instead of a central role for the government and central planning and financing, the presence of small popular groups has come to the fore.

The bottom-up approach to crises is a relatively new field of study that focuses on decentralizing crisis management, enhancing public participation, and mobilizing public resources, which becomes critical during global crises such as pandemics. Given the breadth of this method in Iran's crisis responses and the critical role of (religious) faith as a foundation, the findings of this article can contribute to the growth of the literature in this area. This chapter describes and categorizes a number of initiatives undertaken by these groups during the COVID-19 pandemic: (1) financing, purchasing, and distributing food; (2) public health measures; (3) organizing ceremonies and gatherings; (4) assisting healthcare workers; (5) promptly delivering first time or widely scaled specialized services and products; (6) cultural, promotional, and educational measures; and (7) empowerment of vulnerable, popular actors, and decision makers. This proactive participation of jihadi and civic groups has historically been shaped by the people's collective memory and the centuries-old culture of Help.

Nonetheless, several barriers to this type of crisis response have been identified, including the following: (1) a lack of information; (2) ineffective coordination and cooperation; (3) government dysfunctionality; (4) lack of specialization and learning; and (5) lack of empowerment and provision of root response to needs. These obstacles present opportunities for future research and public actions aimed at improving bottom-up responses to crises.

References

Aldrich, D. P. (2012). *Building resilience: Social capital in post-disaster recovery.* University of Chicago Press.

Bodin, Ö., & Nohrstedt, D. (2016). Formation and performance of collaborative disaster management networks: Evidence *from* a Swedish wildfire response. *Global Environmental Change, 41,* 183–194. https://doi.org/10/f3t26k

Bodin, Ö., Nohrstedt, D., Baird, J., Summers, R., & Plummer, R. (2019). Working at the "speed of trust": Pre-existing and emerging social ties in wildfire responder networks in Sweden and Canada. *Regional Environmental Change, 19*(8), 2353–2364. https://doi.org/10/ghjnhs

Burton, C. G. (2015). A validation of metrics for community resilience to natural hazards and disasters using the recovery *from* Hurricane Katrina as a case study. *Annals of the Association of American Geographers, 105*(1), 67–86. https://doi.org/10/gf7qvw

Chamlee-Wright, E. (2010). *The cultural and political economy of recovery: Social learning in a post-disaster environment.* Routledge.

Cooper, T. L., Bryer, T. A., & Meek, J. W. (2006). Citizen-centered collaborative public management. *Public Administration Review, 66*(s1), 76–88. https://doi.org/10/c42jc8

Correia, P. M. A. R., Mendes, I. de O., Pereira, S. P. M., & Subtil, I. (2020). The Combat against COVID-19 in Portugal, *Part* II: How governance reinforces some organizational values and contributes to the sustainability of crisis management. *Sustainability, 12*(20), 8715. https://doi.org/10/ghj558

Farhadi, M. (2002). *Culture of help in Iran: An introduction to anthropology and sociology of cooperation* (third ed., Vol. 1). Iran University Press (IUP). https://www.gisoom.com/book/1230498/ ‐کتاب‐فرهنگ‐یاریگری‐در‐ایران‐درآمدی‐به‐مردم‐شناسی‐و‐جامعه‐شناسی‐تعاون‐جلد‐1/

French, P. E. (2011). Enhancing the legitimacy of local government pandemic influenza planning through transparency and public engagement. *Public Administration Review, 71*(2), 253–264. https://doi.org/10/fjt3sf

Gallup World Poll. (2020, October 29). *Iranian confidence in government under 50% for first time.* Gallup.Com. https://news.gallup.com/poll/323231/iranian-confidence-government-first-time.aspx

Goulding, C., Kelemen, M., & Kiyomiya, T. (2018). Community based response to the Japanese tsunami: A bottom-up approach. *European Journal of Operational Research, 268*(3), 887–903. https://doi.org/10/ggs7mw

Greyling, C., Maulit, J. A., Parry, S., Robinson, D., Smith, S., Street, A., & Vitillo, R. (2016). Lessons *from* the faith-driven response to the West Africa Ebola epidemic. *The Review of Faith & International Affairs, 14*(3), 118–123. https://doi.org/10/gfhz5r

Grube, L. E. (2020). The what, how, and why of bottom-up rebuilding and recovery after natural disasters. In *Bottom-up Responses to Crisis* (pp. 13–28). Springer.

Grube, L., & Storr, V. H. (2014). The capacity for self-governance and post-disaster resiliency. *The Review of Austrian Economics, 27*(3), 301–324. https://doi.org/10/gkf8r3

Haeffele, S., & Storr, V. H. (Eds.). (2020). *Bottom-up responses to crisis* (1st ed., 2020 edition). Palgrave Macmillan. https://www.amazon.com/Bottom-up-Responses-Mercatus-Studies-Political/dp/3030393119

Hasani Nik, M. A., & Mokhtarianpour, M. (2019). The rationality of jihadi management. *Scientific Journal of Islamic Management, 26*(4), 79–106.

Hayek F. (1945). *The use of knowledge in society, reprinted in: Hayek. FA (1980): Individualism and Economic Order, 77-91.* University of Chicago Press, Chicago, London.

Hurlbert, J. S., Haines, V. A., & Beggs, J. J. (2000). Core networks and tie activation: What kinds of routine networks allocate resources in nonroutine situations? *American Sociological Review, 65*(4), 598–618. https://doi.org/10/bqszk8

Kapucu, N. (2015). Leadership and collaborative governance in managing emergencies and crises. In U. Fra.Paleo (Ed.), *Risk governance* (pp. 211–235). Springer Netherlands. https://doi.org/10.1007/978-94-017-9328-5_13

Kapucu, N., & Ustun, Y. (2018). Collaborative crisis management and leadership in the public sector. *International Journal of Public Administration, 41*(7), 548–561. https://doi.org/10/ghjpkb

Marvi, A., Shahraini, S. M., Yazdi, N., & Maleki, A. (2021). *Iran and COVID-19: A bottom-up, faith-driven, citizen-supported response* [Working paper].

McLennan, B. J. (2020). Conditions for effective coproduction in community-led disaster risk management. *VOLUNTAS: International Journal of Voluntary and Nonprofit Organizations, 31*(2), 316–332. https://doi.org/10.1007/s11266-018-9957-2

Mises, L. V. (1990). *Money, method, and the market process.* Ludwig von Mises Institute.

Paxton, P., & Ressler, R. W. (2018). Trust and participation in associations. In *The Oxford Handbook of Social and Political Trust*, Oxford University Press, Oxford, UK, 149–172.

Penarredonda, J. L. (2020, April 1). Covid-19: The race to build coronavirus ventilators. *BBC.* https://www.bbc.com/future/article/20200401-covid-19-the-race-to-build-coronavirus-ventilators

Pratt, M. G., Lepisto, D. A., & Dane, E. (2018). The hidden side of trust: Supporting and sustaining leaps of faith among firefighters. *Administrative Science Quarterly, 64*(2), 398–434.

Rivera, J. D., & Nickels, A. E. (2014). Social capital, community resilience, and faith-based organizations in disaster recovery: A case study of Mary Queen of Vietnam Catholic Church: A case study of Mary Queen of Vietnam Catholic Church. *Risk, Hazards & Crisis in Public Policy, 5*(2), 178–211. https://doi.org/10/ghjs3f

Storr, V. H., Haeffele-Balch, S., & Grube, L. E. (2016). *Community revival in the wake of disaster: Lessons in local entrepreneurship.* Springer.

Storr, V. H., Haeffele-Balch, S., & Grube, L. E. (2017). Social capital and social learning after Hurricane Sandy. *The Review of Austrian Economics, 30*(4), 447–467. https://doi.org/10/gmnxfs

World Bank. (2017). *Hospital beds (per 1,000 people)—Iran, Islamic Rep. | Data.* World Bank Data. https://data.worldbank.org/indicator/SH.MED.BEDS. ZS?locations=IR

World Bank. (2018). *Physicians (per 1,000 people)—Iran, Islamic Rep. | Data.* World Bank Data. https://data.worldbank.org/indicator/SH.MED.PHYS.ZS? locations=IR

Yamagishi, T., & Yamagishi, M. (1994). Trust and commitment in the United States and Japan. *Motivation and Emotion, 18*(2), 129–166. https://doi.org/10/cwgxdq

Yazdi, N., Marvi, A., & Maleki, A. (2021). Iran and Covid-19: An alternative crisis management system based on bottom-up Islamic social finance and faith-based civic engagement. In *COVID-19 and Islamic Social Finance* (1st ed.). Routledge. https://www.routledge.com/COVID-19-and-Islamic-Social-Finance/ Hassan-Muneeza-Sarea/p/book/9780367639938

Zucker, L. G. (1986). Production of trust: Institutional sources of economic structure, 1840–1920. *Research in Organizational Behavior, 8*, 53–111.

7 Covid-19 and Freedom of Expression in the MENA Region

Alhafad Nouini and Abdelhakim Aboullouz

Introduction

The Covid-19 pandemic is under the spotlight in the scientific and academic communities, being as it is a novel, inexhaustible, and multidimensional field for writing, research, and studies. Covid-19 has caused great upheavals and dilemmas in our contemporary world, as it is perhaps the most dangerous pandemic afflicting humanity over the last century. In the name of protecting their citizens, states have taken remedial and preventive measures.

The Covid-19 pandemic threatens the normal institutional functioning of constitutionally governed states, and it threatens the lives of persons residing in these states. There looms fear of a large death toll from the pandemic. This rare, exceptional state of affairs has required urgent, unusual, and exceptional measures, foremost among them a state of emergency. A state of emergency is declared to run and protect the country, in accordance with the famous Roman saying "The safety of the People is above the law" (Abdelkarim, 2008). Seemingly overnight, states of emergencies were adopted all over the world, impelling us to review the concept of the state of emergency together with related or equivalent concepts, such as the state of exception, the state of health emergency, and the state of siege. These states all refer to legal systems that replace the normal functioning of a country's system of governance (Janjin, 2020). In particular, a state of emergency leads to the expansion of a government's executive powers and its security institutions, as security apparatuses are primarily in charge of governing during extraordinary or exceptional times. Concurrently, the state of emergency shrinks the space to exercise rights and freedoms in a country.

The concept of a state of emergency, siege, or exception was linked in earlier times to military coups against the ruling regimes. As such, a state of emergency is usually correlated with a security disruption or attempt at regime change. With few exceptions, a state of emergency has never before been associated with a public health crisis. This includes but is not limited to the 'Spanish Flu' (Nouini, 2020) in 1918, the SARS virus afflicting China and other countries in 2002–2003 (Reladunes, 2020), the swine flu in 2009, and the Ebola virus, which had two outbreaks in 1976 and 2014

DOI: 10.4324/9781003266259-7

(Soliman, 2020). Now a public health crisis has arrived in the form of Covid-19, which is responsible for the most widespread public health emergency as of yet witnessed on a global scale in the twenty-first century.

This chapter highlights an important aspect of the Covid-19 crisis, which is the impact of the state of emergency declarations in Morocco and Tunisia on basic rights and freedoms, especially the right to free expression and opinion. By studying and monitoring the impact of these emergency declarations on human rights in the two countries, this chapter confirms the hypothesis that Morocco and Tunisia took advantage of the state of emergency, using it not only to confront Covid-19 but also to extend and reinforce their regimes' security reach and authoritarianism at the expense of rights and freedoms. Setbacks have resulted in rights victories achieved after the 2011 uprisings in the MENA region. These rights are stipulated in the two recent constitutions of Morocco and Tunisia, enacted in 2011 and 2014, respectively, especially the right to freedom of opinion and expression.

The main question problematized by this chapter is the extent to which the state of emergency impacted rights and freedoms in Morocco and Tunisia, especially the right to freedom of opinion and expression. In order to problematize this question, this chapter relies on the analytical legal method, which is based on analysing and deconstructing legal, regulatory, and constitutional texts to reach conclusions on concepts, expressed through the texts, within the context in which they were written. The case study method will also be used as an analytical tool.

State of Emergency in the International System, Rights and Freedoms

The study of the state of emergency is important, albeit the enactment of an emergency state hypothetically only occurs in exceptional circumstances and in specific contexts and for specific durations of time. In other words, the state of emergency is framed with conditions that temporally limit its field of action. During states of emergency or exception, a departure from the ordinary happens, which, in turn, limits a number of rights and freedoms stipulated in international charters and national constitutions.

The definitions of the state of emergency differ between a number of thinkers, researchers, and writers, rendering it difficult to accurately define and categorise. French jurist Maurice Horio defined the state of emergency as 'a legal system prepared in advance to secure the country, based on strengthening powers by transferring civilian power to the hands of the military authority' (Al-Chourabi and Jadallah, 2020).

Yazilian Kensch defined it as:

> the state that occurs when exceptional crises and disturbances are provoked, and can be considered a legal system in the service of the state, which meets the requirements of efficiency in the context of war or

crisis, and which uses methods of restraint to maintain public order. These legal techniques must enable the state to achieve the goal it seeks to achieve – i.e., the rule of law – especially by concentrating the powers in its hand and restricting rights and freedoms.

When reviewing the definitions of the state of emergency, we note that most of them fall short of providing a direct definition, instead limiting themselves to presenting the purpose of the state of emergency's declaration. In general, the purpose of a state of emergency is to strengthen the executive authority by transferring some of the legislative and judicial powers to it, or to establish an exceptional legal system for the benefit of the institutions of the executive authority. The latter is liberated from the restrictions imposed on it during ordinary circumstances. In addition, the exercise of a number of rights and freedoms is restricted under the state of emergency's cover, to a degree that sometimes exceeds acceptable limits (Jamil, 1963). The state of emergency is referenced in international law, within international agreements. International human rights treaties have granted states the right to place restrictions on the exercise of internationally guaranteed rights, as these treaties are the legal basis for declaring a state of emergency in exceptional circumstances. The International Covenant on Civil and Political Rights (ICCPR), and the International Covenant on Economic, Social and Cultural Rights (ICESCR) include provisions that allow member states to restrict rights and freedoms under their national laws in a state of emergency.

International human rights law regulates how this power is exercised so that it does not become an excuse that the state can freely use and so that the emergency declaration is decided upon according to its own merits and practices. International human rights law has established a legal system for rights restrictions in normal and exceptional circumstances, to ensure that human rights abuses and violations do not occur and to ensure the legitimacy of restricting rights and freedoms is enshrined in national legislation (Abdulqadir, 2012). The ICCPR regulates the practice and restriction of political and civil rights during a state of emergency. The ICCPR is the basic rights convention included within the framework of the United Nations. Outside of the UN framework, the right to free expression is guaranteed by both the European and American conventions on human rights, while this right is not guaranteed by the African Charter on Human and Peoples' Rights (Ouguergouz, 1994).

States and governments have begun to respect the rules and ethics underlying the declaration of an exceptional or emergency state, since it was stipulated in the ICCPR, which entered into force on 23 March 1976. Article 4 of the ICCPR provides for the conditions necessitating the practice of an emergency state and for restriction upon the exercise of fundamental rights and freedoms (ICCPR, 1976). In addition to the ICCPR, there are European Convention on Human Rights and the American Convention on

Human Rights, which entered into force in 1958 and 1978 respectively (IC-CPR, 1976). The conventions address the state of emergency and restrictions on the exercise of some rights under emergency circumstances and the conditions for deploying these restrictions. There are also the Siracusa Principles of 1984, adopted by the United Nations Social and Economic Council, as well as the general comments issued by the Human Rights Committee. These principles, developed by a committee of 21 international experts, provide guidance on the state of emergency and rights and freedoms. Explanations are given for all measures that may be taken in the context of the state of emergency and in regard to restricting fundamental rights and freedoms (ICCPR, 1976). When declaring a state of emergency, international law stipulates conditions that must be met to restrict rights and freedoms:

- Threatening the life of the nation. What is meant by this criterion is that the state party to the International Covenant is exposed to an imminent and unusual danger, which necessitates the disavowal of its international obligations arising from it, especially in the field of human rights. This disavowal of obligations, including human rights obligations, is deemed necessary due to the extraordinary circumstances threatening the state's existence and stability, which, in turn, impedes the functioning of public life within it, jeopardising the entire nation;
- Official declaration. The state is required to officially declare the state of emergency;
- The goal of this declaration shall be to protect public interest;
- Determining the period of time and achieving balance. The state must achieve a balance when it limits rights and freedoms during a state of exception and emergency – a balance between the measures and procedures it takes during this period and the requirements of the situation within the limits of the state of emergency, provided that the conditions are met for declaring a state of emergency and for restricting the exercise of the rights stipulated in the International Covenant;
- Legal stipulation. That is, this situation must be stipulated in the domestic law of the state – especially the constitution – so that all its procedures are constitutional and legal.
- Rights that may not be suspended. Article 4 of the ICCPR stipulated the right of states to suspend fundamental rights and freedoms, by providing conditions in normal and exceptional circumstances for the permissibility of this restriction. In the same article, in the second paragraph, it excluded some of the stipulated rights in Articles 6 and 7, the first and second paragraphs of Article 8, as well as Articles 11, 15, and 16, of this restriction. This is because the rights contained within these articles are not subject to infringement, and the state is prohibited from including them in the rights that are subject to suspension. These rights are protected by the force of international law and therefore they cannot be abandoned, in order to preserve human dignity in all circumstances by the state parties to the International Covenant (ICCPR, 1976).

In general, it appears that the provisions of Article 4 (that prohibit the state from excluding or violating the fundamental rights referred to in the second paragraph during a state of emergency) did not achieve the goal for which these provisions were stipulated. Imposing restrictions or limiting other rights related to the inviolable rights made the latter rights to have little effect when declaring a state of public emergency in the country.

On the other hand, the obligation of state parties under the third paragraph of Article 4 to inform other state parties immediately of the provisions to which they did not adhere and the reasons that prompted them to do so, is intended to circumscribe the powers of the state when it restricts or denies basic rights. In this respect, Article 4 establishes a system for international monitoring of the extent to which the state respects fundamental rights and freedoms, during normal or exceptional circumstances (Al-Awadi, 1984). According to international law, the state of emergency is an exceptional state that cannot be transformed into a normal state of governance that lasts indefinitely. Neither can it be used by governments as a cover to restrict and disrupt the exercise of the fundamental rights and freedoms guaranteed by international human rights conventions and contained within the constitutions of most countries (Khamous, 2008).

Legal Framing of Covid-19's State of Emergency in Morocco and Tunisia

Most national constitutions frame states of exception and emergency in a way that gives public authorities more powers to manage the situation. In connection with the Covid-19 pandemic, a health crisis afflicting the world, most countries did not differentiate between the state of emergency and the state of health emergency in their legal systems. They consider the latter as a rare occurrence, so it is absent from their legal systems. In contrast, there commonly is a legal and constitutional framing for the state of emergency. Furthermore, there are also countries that have adopted a state of health emergency. Accordingly, we will refer to the state of emergency and the state of health emergency as one state – simply a state of emergency – since the first includes the second.

In the case of Morocco, the government attempted to respond to the standards stipulated in international law. As such, the Moroccan Constitution of 2011 stipulated a state of exception and emergency in Articles 59 and 74, to give the king broad powers to take measures by way of adapting to changing emergency circumstances. These include the power to suspend the exercise of rights and freedoms. By indicating the parameters of the exceptional circumstances, Morocco's constitution has adhered to the basic standard stipulated in the ICCPR, especially with regard to threats to territorial integrity, or the occurrence of events that hinder the normal functioning of government institutions (Al-Awadi, 1984).

The reasons necessitating the declaration of a state of exception according to the 2011 Moroccan Constitution are broad and vague. The language is malleable and imprecise, which leaves the interpretation of constitutional provisions open to the ruling authority, which may consider virtually anything a threat to territorial integrity or an obstruction upon the functioning of public institutions (Robert, 1993). Consequently, the interpretation remains open to events during which the authority may deem it necessary to declare a state of exception, which in some cases may not constitute a real threat to the nation's territorial integrity or the functioning of its institutions (Al-Fahri, 1999).

The Moroccan government had previously declared a state of exception and emergency, but it was largely due to an explicit threat to the ruling system. Moroccan constitutions thus sought to grant absolute authority to the executive government authorities, in regard to determining the reasons for declaring a national state of emergency. A debate arose on this issue after King Hassan II declared a state of exception in 1965, which confirmed the orientation of the Moroccan constitutions regarding emergency/exception (Rabi'I, 2013). All this left the Kingdom in a legal and constitutional vacuum when it was hit by the global health crisis of Covid-19. This pushed the government to rectify the matter by stipulating Decree Law No. 2.20.292 related to the state of health emergency and the procedures for declaring it, and Decree No. 2.20.293 related to declaring a state of health emergency across the country to confront the coronavirus outbreak (Tabih, 2020). The Moroccan government invoked Article 81 of the constitution, which allows it to issue laws during the interval between parliamentary sessions (Tabih, 2020).

The two decrees – consisting of seven articles in the first and five in the second – declared that Morocco is in a state of health emergency under Article 1 of Decree Law No. 2.20.292. That decree also affirmed that the government has the right to take all legislative, organisational, administrative and other measures during the emergency period. It deemed it within the government's powers to mobilise all possible means and measures necessary to prevent the Covid-19 crisis from worsening (Official Gazette, 2020), whereas Article 4 of the same decree states that anyone who violates orders and decisions issued by the public authorities is subject to imprisonment for a duration ranging from one to three months and a fine ranging from 300 to 1,300 Moroccan dirhams (28 to 121 euros). This is in addition to the application of the penal code or criminal law when deemed necessary. The article adds that all citizens are subject to the same penalty if they obstruct or interfere with – in any manner – the work of the public authorities in managing emergency or exceptional circumstances (Official Gazette, 2020).

The Moroccan government, in Decree No. 2.20.293 related to the procedures for declaring a state of health emergency, defined these measures and determined their duration (set them for 30 days). It generally stipulated the transfer of all legislative, executive and administrative powers in favour of the Ministry of Interior and authority figures, from governors, workers and leaders subordinate on various local scales. This decree enabled them to take all measures and issue any decision required by the state of health emergency, in a way that gives Ministry of Interior officials the power to enact these measures based on their personal reading of the epidemiological situation in the geographical areas in which they are based. The measures taken were related to movement in general, as the right to movement was prohibited with few exceptions by means of a travel permit granted by the Ministry of Interior's local officials (Official Gazette, 2020). The government did not stop at the two decrees. It continued to extend the state of health emergency by legislating new decrees without resorting to parliament, which is invested with original jurisdiction. In 2020, the government issued Decree No. 2.20.330 on 9 April, Decree No. 2.20.371 dated 19 May, Decree No. 2.20. 406 dated 9 June and Decree No. 2.20.503 dated 8 August (Official Gazette, 2020).

The legislation of all these decrees sparked an extensive debate in academic, partisan and political circles inside Morocco, given that the government did not find direct constitutional support for the decrees, and relied on articles 21, 24, and 81. Intensifying the debate was the executive governing authority's lack of reliance on parliament, and its failure to involve parliament in other decrees. Nevertheless, there remain legislative solutions to deal with the legal vacuum related to the state of emergency. In this chapter, we focus on rights and freedoms during this period, without entering into debates related to the legal and constitutional framework regulating the state of emergency in Morocco.

In comparison, the Tunisian state has witnessed less debate and disagreement than Morocco in regard to the legal and constitutional framework regulating the state of emergency. This is because Tunisia has been under a state of emergency since late 2015, after the terrorist attack on the presidential security convoy in the capital Tunis (Al-Thabity, 2020). Since then, the state of emergency has remained declared in Tunisia, renewed every time. When the pandemic reached Tunisia, the legal basis for taking favourable measures had already been established, given that the country was already in a state of emergency. Executive decisions and orders were straightforward to issue. President Kais Saied, by presidential order, imposed curfew all over Tunisia from 6 p.m. to 8 a.m., starting on 18 March 2020 until further notice, with exceptions made for medical emergencies (Decaf, 2020). The President issued a second order, in the context of responding to Covid-19, that banned gatherings of more than three persons in public places. It banned the movement of people and vehicles during curfew times (Decaf, 2020). The presidential orders, similar to decrees, are legally binding and constitutionally based, especially Article 80 of the constitution, which gives the president the right to enact measures necessitated by the state of emergency (Decaf, 2020). The Tunisian state also granted a mandate to the head of government in the form Law 19 of 2020, whereby the president can issue legislative decrees to confront and address the Covid-19 pandemic. This law, which consists of four articles, covers rights and freedoms. It provides that the management of human rights in Tunisia during a state of emergency will be in line with the epidemiological situation in the country. The law contains provisions on how to resist the spread of the virus and harness efforts to eradicate it, in a manner that does not contradict the requirements of Article 49 of the Tunisian Constitution (Decaf, 2020).

In the same context, and in order to control the spread of the pandemic, the Tunisian government criminalised every breach of curfew during quarantine and set a fine for those who violate the curfew at 50 Tunisian dinars (fifteen and a half euros). Furthermore, anyone (especially the infected) who does not comply with the preventive and remedial measures to limit the spread of the novel coronavirus is penalised with a fine ranging from 1,000 to 5,000 Tunisian dinars (308 and 1544 euros). In the event that a person is the source of transmission to another person, the vector shall be punished according to the criminal procedures law and the penal code, as the vector is considered a person who has committed a crime requiring imprisonment (Al-Rayed Al-Rasmy, 2020a). Based on that law, the government issued another decree to address the social and economic impacts of the coronavirus. According to the decree, the quarantine is to be gradually lifted in accordance with a strict preventive system, and some economic activities can be resumed according to a specific program and government plan related to developments and evaluation of the pandemic situation in the country (GCSSG, 2020). In July, the Prime Minister issued a government order to end the state of comprehensive quarantine imposed on the country during the month of March 2020 (Al-Rayed Al-Rasmy, 2020a). The state of emergency continued and was extended for six months, beginning on 30 May 2020 and ending on 25 November 2020, by order of the President who had previously stated that the emergency law is unconstitutional, saying that he is, 'obliged to extend the state of emergency, like someone holding a burning coal' (Al-Rayed Al-Rasmy, 2020b). There were many violations of rights and freedoms during the state of emergency in Tunisia, and these violations were shown even more clearly during the imposition of the quarantine. There was a debate regarding the constitutionality of the presidential order of 2015 declaring a state of emergency in the country, which continued to extend automatically; there was also debate regarding the legality of restrictions on the exercise of some rights. Article 49 in the constitution explicitly provides that: 'The law determines the controls related to the rights and freedoms guaranteed in this constitution and their exercise in a way that does not undermine their essence' (Al-Rayed Al-Rasmy, 2014).

Impact of the Health Emergency on Freedom of Expression in Morocco and Tunisia

Restricting freedoms under the pretext of applying the law has been problematic throughout history. For example, the US Supreme Court heard a case in 1985 on the killing of a child, accused of stealing ten dollars, by a policeman during pursuit (Tennesse Caring, 1985). Several issues were raised.

Although the policeman behaved according to the law and sought to preserve public order, that behaviour cost a person's life over a very small sum of money. Is it permissible to deprive a person of their right to life in order to preserve public order, security or health? Does the problem lie within the laws that do not provide for the principle of proportionality and gradualism in the strict application of the legal rule across different contexts? (Al-Majry, 2018). The Office of the United Nations High Commissioner for Human Rights has warned against the exploitation of states of emergency by governments to retreat from human rights gains. The OHCHR called for the observance and inclusion of human rights during the response to Covid-19, and a number of United Nations human rights experts issued a memorandum at the beginning of the pandemic's global spread, in which they warned countries against using state of emergency to settle scores with individuals or groups, or to suppress and violate human rights in their countries (Al-Majry, 2020). Since their respective declarations of a state of emergency in response to the Covid-19 pandemic, both Morocco and Tunisia have taken a number of measures that restrict the rights and freedoms of their citizens. While many rights were negatively affected during the public health crisis, the focus of this study is limited to freedom of expression and opinion, as an illustrative case. In Morocco, since the declaration of the state of emergency and the restriction of movement throughout the country on 20 March 2020, all powers have been transferred to the executive authority, and the hand of the Ministry of the Interior has been significantly extended ever since, especially in regard to violating rights and freedoms. A large number of the executive authority's agents have transgressed human rights, and at times, cases of violence by security forces against citizens, especially in the first weeks of the health emergency, were documented (Najdy, 2020).

The Moroccan government also took advantage of the exceptional global health emergency to restrict and deny the right to free expression and opinion in the country. It prevented the printing of newspapers for more than two months and did not allow printing to resume until 26 May 2020 (Abdulsamad, 2020). Moroccan human rights organisations considered the Moroccan authorities' violations of the right to free expression during the health emergency as tantamount to a 'human rights setback'. Within the framework of Law Decree No. 2.20.292, the Public Prosecutor's Office moved the arrest and prosecution of 91,623 persons who violated the state of emergency, including 558 people in detention simply for violating quarantine measures, up to 22 May 2020 – according to an official statement from the Moroccan Public Prosecution Office (Public Ministry, 2020). Among the detainees were five journalists arrested solely for exercising their right to free expression and opinion. After expressing their views on the state's response to the Covid-19 crisis, the journalists were arrested and prosecuted under emergency law on charges such as 'broadcasting false facts', which does not constitute a crime in such exceptional circumstances, according to the international standards (Public Ministry, 2020). Three journalists from among the five arrested – Mohamed Bouzrou, Mohamed Shajia and Hassan Al-Morabti – were arrested on 17 and 19 April for expressing their opinions on a Facebook page called 'Fazaz 24'. They criticised some of the government's behaviours and actions in regard to measures taken in response to the Covid-19 crisis. This included a comment about the 'clientelism' that marred the distribution of aid to citizens. Later on, the authorities released one of the journalists, while the other two remain behind bars (Public Ministry, 2020). On 15 May, security forces arrested another journalist in the city of Figuig because he too exercised his natural right to express his opinion, which is guaranteed by all international covenants and Morocco's 2011 constitution. Authorities arrested the journalist after he commented on social media that he considers some practices by authority figures to be 'violations of human rights'. Amna Goulali, Deputy Director of the Middle East and North Africa Regional Office at Amnesty International, said that Morocco should not use the state of emergency to 'silence the voices of those who dare to criticize the government's measures to confront and deal with the pandemic' (Public Ministry, 2020).

The Moroccan government further exploited the state of emergency by attempting to pass law number 22.20 related to the use of social networks. The law was set to restrict freedom of opinion and expression for Moroccan citizens, especially on social networks (Azzam, 2020). Yet, the law's passage was prevented by the pressure exerted by Moroccan public opinion, including a substantial amount of popular protest and rejection on social media, forcing the government to postpone its consideration (Ghabshi, 2020). The law, which was presented by the Minister of Justice and approved by the Government Council, is evidence of the concerns previously raised about the exploitation of the state of emergency to eliminate basic rights and freedoms, foremost among them the right to freedom of opinion and expression.

The 'postponed' bill consists of 25 articles, including articles that criminalise speech on the Internet. Article 14 stipulates that anyone who incites a boycott of products, goods or services shall be punished with imprisonment of three months to three years and a fine of 5,000 to 50,000 Moroccan dirhams. Article 16 of the draft law itself criminalises anyone who publishes or promotes electronic content, which includes false news, with a prison sentence of three months to two years and a fine of 1,000 to 5,000 Moroccan dirhams (Al-Nasry, 2020). It is worth noting here that the falsity of the news is determined by the government, and therefore there is no specific and clear criterion for determining the meaning of 'falsity' here. The articles of this law contradict international human rights obligations, and in particular the article 19 of the ICCPR, which does not allow states to restrict freedom of opinion and expression except in accordance with international standards. Accordingly, the United Nations ranked Morocco among the countries that violated human rights during the state of emergency to confront Covid-19. The Office of the High Commissioner for Human Rights confirmed in a statement that there are more than 80 countries – including Morocco – that have exploited the state of emergency to violate rights and freedoms while citing the need to resolve the public health crisis. The High Commissioner's statement stressed that, 'emergency powers must not be transformed into a weapon in the hands of governments to be used against opposition, monitor peoples and stay in power' (Alif Post, 2020). The rights situation in Tunisia is less severe compared to Morocco. Since its announcement of the quarantine to confront the outbreak of the novel coronavirus, the government has taken a number of measures and procedures, the first of which was to impose a curfew on 18 March 2020 and tighten the screws on people's freedoms outside the hours of the ban. The President used the army – deployed on the national level across the territory – to impose these measures under the cover of fighting the pandemic's spread (Garrad, 2020). Several Tunisian human rights organisations confirmed that these governmental measures were taken to limit the right of citizens to express opinions on public policies in the country, taking advantage of the quarantine. Rights organisations also condemned the arbitrary practices of security personnel against individuals who left their homes for shopping. The Tunisian authorities took advantage of the state of emergency and quarantine imposed in the country due to the Covid-19 pandemic and arrested a Tunisian blogger simply for expressing her opinion. The blogger in question shared a satirical post on her Facebook page entitled 'Surat Corona'. She was sentenced to six months imprisonment and a fine of 2,000 dinars (616 euros) for 'insulting the sacred, outraging morals and inciting violence'. Human rights organisations, including Amnesty International, called for the release of the Tunisian blogger and for the government to respect free opinion and expression, especially considering Tunisia's status as an emerging democracy in which it is not appropriate for the government to exploit a public health emergency to restrict basic freedoms and rights (DW, 2020).

Tunisian rights activists are concerned about the rapidity with which this blogger's case was handled. Some expressed astonishment at the way the case proceeded, especially in light of the exceptional circumstances in Tunisia – the state of emergency and quarantine. What raised suspicion is that the authorities did not prosecute more serious violations, such as domestic violence, in the same speed and manner (Badri, 2020). This is even more problematic given that Tunisia's 2014 constitution – considered the most supreme legal document in the country – guarantees the exercise of freedom of opinion and expression for all individuals without restriction. Media professionals and those interested in Tunisian public affairs expressed their dismay and frustration at the measures taken by the government under the cover of the health emergency and home quarantine, which contributed to restricting freedoms and hindering access to information. In effect, official media platforms became the only parties that obtained information, which, in turn, made the exploitation and manipulation of this information highly probable. On the occasion of World Press Freedom Day, Ritaj Ibrahim of the Arab Foundation for Freedoms and Equality stated: 'This pandemic has placed additional restrictions and made the task of journalists more difficult, as it made it difficult for them to access information, and complete information cannot be accessed through the use of the Internet only' (AFE, 2020). Tunisia continues to exploit the state of emergency and quarantine to restrict rights and freedoms, especially free expression and opinion. It is still unwilling to legislate a law regulating the press council, which, in turn, would ensure the protection of freedom of expression and the press from deviations, abuses of power, and unprofessional practices by the authorities. A law regulating the Press Council would develop a code of ethics based on respect for human rights and free expression, contributing to education on human rights in Tunisian society, given that genuine democracies value a free press. The Tunisian government, however, is still hindering the process, and during the home quarantine period withdrew a bill on the press council (Baghori, 2020). On the legislative front, Tunisia exploited the state of emergency to make urgent amendments to articles 245 and 247 of the Criminal Code, with the aim of controlling free opinion on social networks and restricting free expression in all electronic media, criminalising the '[disclosure of] any false or suspicious speech among users of social media networks and platforms, which may be offensive to individuals, groups, or institutions' (Global Voice, 2020). These amendments regarding freedom of expression in the digital sphere completely contravene the Tunisian constitution and international human rights obligations. Article 31 of the constitution guarantees the freedom of expression, thought, opinion and access to information. It affirms that censorship is not permissible, while Article 49 states that the law defines the controls and restrictions on rights and freedoms in a manner that does not affect their essence and adds that no amendment is permissible that contradicts human rights gains guaranteed in the constitution. Nevertheless, Tunisia's violations of free expression and opinion during the state of emergency remain less severe than Morocco's violations. The latter recorded a large number of cases in which the right to free expression, thought and opinion was restricted. In general, all Arab countries, especially in North Africa, have taken advantage of the state of emergency declared during Covid-19 to limit the exercise of rights and freedoms. In particular, states sought to control freedom of expression and settle their accounts with dissidents during this exceptional period. This should not be the case, given that these countries are undergoing extraordinary circumstances that require a focus on overcoming the crisis rather than making gains for regimes. Countries must rely on UN and international standards when dealing with human rights during pandemics, crises, emergencies, and exceptional circumstances, to allow their citizens to discuss and debate issues related to home quarantine, as well as express their views on measures and procedures related to public health emergencies. Previous experience with HIV showed that there is no justification for restricting and limiting rights and freedoms, especially free expression and access to information. On the contrary, systems must be in place to guarantee access to information and to allow everyone to freely express opinions and ideas (UNAIDS, 2020).

Conclusion

The Covid-19 pandemic has demonstrated the fragility and weakness of constitutional guarantees for rights and freedoms in North African countries, including those countries caught in the fervour of the 2011 Arab uprisings and that developed and changed their constitutions in consideration of international human rights standards. Likewise, the pandemic made clear that authoritarian regimes always remain true to their authoritarian traditions; they need only an opportunity to reproduce the same old authoritarian patterns. This is what we observed in the cases of Morocco and Tunisia, which witnessed multiple violations of rights and freedoms – especially the right to free opinion and expression – during the state of emergency enveloping the two countries. Government authorities in Morocco and Tunisia arrested journalists and citizens simply for expressing their views and also attempted to restrict this right by legislating draconian laws. This highlights the importance of having constitutional provisions and legal texts regulating the right to freedom of expression, opinion and thought, formulated in a way that fully recognises this fundamental right in the democratic system. This legislation should ensure that the exercise of rights is not subject to restrictions set during exceptional circumstances except in a clear manner that evokes proportionality and the Siracusa Principles in detail and free of any ambiguity and confusion that can be exploited by states. Yet, in Morocco and Tunisia – two constitutional states that have stipulated their commitment to international rights standards – the violation of human rights is the norm, not the exception. This widespread lack of respect for rights in the two countries was made evident in the context of their respective declarations of an emergency state in response to Covid-19. Both states took advantage of this period to consolidate the authoritarianism of their security apparatuses and to grant the executive ruling authority more powers against all other branches of governance.

References

Abdelkarim, Faris Hamed (2008) 'Safety of the people is above the law: the doctrine of constitutional transcendence and the theory of needs in hard times for the state', Al-Nour, 21 February, accessed 11 August 2020, https://bit.ly/3kuL1N7

Abdulqadir, Laraj (2012) PhD thesis, Morocco, p. 182.

Abdulsamad, Mohamed (2020) 'Morocco, Corona adds to the plights of paper journalism', Anatolia, 2 July, accessed 25 August 2020, https://bit.ly/3ltr8P2

AFE (2020) 'Press freedom and the coronavirus,' Arab Foundation for Freedoms and Equality, 3 May, accessed 27 August 2020, https://bit.ly/31xAEQY

Al-Awadi, Badriya (1984) 'Provisions restricting basic human rights in the ICCPR and constitutions of the Gulf states', *Gulf Studies Journal*, vol 10/40, p. 30.

Al-Chourabi, Abdulhamid and Sherif Jadallah (2000) 'The prospects of unconstitutionality and illegitimacy of the decisions to declare and extend state of emergency and military control', Egypt: Munsha'a Al-Maarif, p. 44.

Al-Fahri, Al-Fasi Youssif (1999) 'International human rights law in the constitutions of North Africa', PhD Thesis, Rabat: Legal, Economic and Social Sciences, University of Aghdal, 1998/1999, p. 138.

Al-Majry, Karim (2020) 'The problematic relationship between state of emergency stipulations for Covid-19 and human rights and freedoms, in International law', Al-Jazeera Center for Human Rights and Freedoms, accessed 24 August 2020, https://bit.ly/3hxn460

Al-Majry, Khaled (2018) 'Restrictions and rules for rights and freedoms: comment on article 41 of the Tunisian Constitution', Tunisia: The International Institution for Elections and Democracy Publications, p. 7.

Al-Nasry, Nouraldin (2020) Reading the bill number 22.20 regarding the use of social networks, open networks and the like, 10 May, accessed 26 August 2020, https://bit.ly/32rgoQh

Al-Rayed Al-Rasmy (2014) Tunisian constitution, 10 February 2014.

Al-Rayed Al-Rasmy (2020a) Governmental order 411/2020 dated 3 July 2020 regarding lifting the comprehensive quarantine and stopping some governmental orders, number 156/2020, dated 22 March 2020, regarding the provision of basic needs and the requirements of the continuation of vital infrastructure in the context of applying comprehensive quarantine (2020), accessed 22 August 2020, https://bit.ly/31nbYLa

Al-Rayed Al-Rasmy (2020b) Law 19/2020, dated 12 April 2020, regarding mandating the head of the government to issue decrees to face the consequences of the Coronavirus situation (2020). Al-Rayed Al-Rasmy, vol 31, dated 12 April 2020.

Al-Thabity, Adel (2020) 'Tunisia... extending the state of emergency 6 months', Anatolia Press, 29 May, accessed 22 August 2020, https://bit.ly/31ppY7f

Alif Post (2020) 'UN ranks Morocco among states that committed violations in the context of coronavirus related emergency', Alef Post, 29 April, accessed 26 August 2020, https://bit.ly/2CZYyLw

Azzam, Ismail (2020) 'Why did the bill on social networks cause widespread anger in Morocco?' DW, 29 April, accessed 26 August, https://bit.ly/3hylrES

Badri, Fatima (2020) 'In Tunisia: no freedom of expression against the "sacred"', Daraj al-Ikhbari, 3 June, accessed 27 August 2020, https://bit.ly/31x5clX

Baghori, Nagi (2020) 'Freedom of expression challenged!' Nawah, 4 May, accessed 27 August 2020, https://bit.ly/31yLA0F

DECAF (2020) Presidential order 24/2020 issued 18 March 2020 regarding curfew across the republic (2020) Geneva Center for Security Sector Governance, 18 March, accessed 22 August, https://bit.ly/3j2fel5

DW (2020) 'Tunisia: blogger imprisoned after sharing a satirical post, "Sourat Corona"', DW, 14 July, accessed 27 August 2020, https://bit.ly/3lodQel

Garrad, Aya (2020) 'Tunisia faces the corona procedures: exceptional measures to confront exceptional circumstances?' Paris: Arab Reform Initiative, April 2020, p. 3.

GCSSG (2020) Decree issued by head of the government, number 9/2020 dated 17 April 2020, regarding confronting violation of curfew and comprehensive quarantine and procedures for persons suspected of being infected by Covid-19 (2020). Geneva Center for Security Sector Governance, 17 April 2020, accessed 22 August 2020, https://bit.ly/3hqYx2g

Ghabshi, Bualam (2020) 'Did the Moroccan government dismiss the social networks law because of popular anger?' France 24, 5 May, accessed 29 October 2020, https://bit.ly/3hylrES

Global Voice (2020) 'Impact of coronavirus containment measures on the human rights and civil freedoms movement in MENA', Global Voice, 13 April, accessed 27 August 2020, https://bit.ly/31wPp6L

ICCPR (1976) OHCHR | International covenant on civil and political rights. United Nations Human Rights. https://www.ohchr.org/en/professionalinterest/pages/ccpr.aspx

Jamil, Hussien (1963) Martial orders, Baghdad, p. 64.

Janjin, Al-Hussien Mohamed (2020) 'Legitimacy of restricting human rights during health crises', Maroc Doura, 18 May, accessed 11 August 2020, https://bit.ly/3gOE3Qx

Khamous, Amr Abdulla (2008) 'Impact of emergency law on individual freedoms in constitutions', Kurdistan Strategic Studies Publications, p. 57.

Najdy, Adel (2020) 'Emergency in Morocco raises concerns about rights violations', Al-Arabi al-Jadid, 31 March, accessed 25 August 2020, https://bit.ly/31sGYcH

Nouini, Elhafad (2020) 'Impact of Covid-19 on freedom of expression in Morocco and Tunisia', Rowaq Arabi 25 (4), pp. 33–48.

Official Gazette, vol 6874, 25 Shaban 1441 (19 April 2020), p. 2218.

Ouguergouz, F (1994) 'L'absence de clause de dérogation dans certains traités relatifs aux droits de l'homme: les réponses du droit international générale', p. 291.

Public Ministry (2020) Statement about violations of the state of health emergency, 22 May, Public Prosecution Office of Morocco, accessed 25 August 2020, https://bit.ly/3aWYk4D

Rabi'I, Hamid (2013) 'Status of international treaties in the new constitution: the case of international human rights treaties', Moroccan Journal for Local Administration and Development 82 Rabat, p. 403.

Reladunes, Timas, translated by Nawar (2020) 'The gravest pandemics in history', Fossils, 2 April, accessed 29 October 2020, https://bit.ly/35JfXm5

Robert, Jacque (1993) 'L'état de l'exception dans la constitution du Maroc, dans Trente années de vie constitutionnelle au Maroc', p. 244.

Soliman, Amer (2020) 'The deadliest pandemics across history: how did the world face them?' TRT Arabic, 25 March, accessed 29 October 2020, https://bit.ly/35K1Kb5

Tabih, Abdulkabir (2020) 'The need for applying article 81 of the Constitution', Al-Awal, 21 March, accessed 21 August 2020, https://bit.ly/3l8Orp9

Tennesse Caring (1985) Decision 471, US Supreme Court, dated 17 March, Washington.

UNAIDS (2020) 'Rights in the time of Covid-19', The Joint United Nations Programme on HIV and AIDS, Switzerland, Geneva, 2020, p. 8.

8 Policy Responses to Covid-19 Pandemic in the Maghreb Region

Hamid Ait El Caid

Introduction

As of June 1, 2021, more than 170 million cases have been reported across 188 countries and territories, resulting in more than 3.5 million deaths.[1] The Covid-19 pandemic has created a tremendous state of panic and disorder in the world. Almost all countries took urgent measures to stop the spread of the disease which were not only limited to healthcare system but were extended to all sectors of government. For instance, Italy and Spain which were among the first, most affected countries with high number of infection and fatality cases tightened measures to counter the spread of the virus and slow its speed through total lockdown and restriction of movement. Not far from Spain and Italy, The Maghreb, comprising of Algeria, Morocco and Tunisia, recorded the first confirmed infection of Covid-19 in Algeria on February 25, 2020. In the course of March of the same year, more cases have been recorded in the three countries, which forced the respective governments to start immediate actions related to lockdown, in addition to other measures concerning health and epidemiological situation, as well as measures addressing socio-economic consequences.

This chapter seeks to assess the Covid-19 policy responses in the Maghreb. Thus, the assessment model adopted in this study is "program evaluation" which is centered around five key domains: needs assessment; program theory and design; program process; program impact; and program efficiency.[2]

Needs assessment: an important factor leading to the decision of program evaluation is the need to alleviate a social problem of public concern. The latter can be recognized as an issue undermining social development, such as poverty, unemployment or education efficiency, while other issues may trigger the national economy such as inflation, recession and budget deficit. Another issue that requires policy action is the health situation in cases of epidemics, infectious diseases and pandemics such as Covid-19. Pointing to this research, Covid-19 pandemic presents a crucial problem that demands the need to intervene, because it puts people's health and life at risk as well as their social stability conditions as a result of lockdown and closure of businesses. Thus, needs for policy intervention due to health situation and

DOI: 10.4324/9781003266259-8

socio-economic consequences are addressed in the context of the Maghreb states' anti-Covid-19 measures.

Program theory and design: after a problem is recognized and its needs for policy actions are identified, now it is up to the policymakers to design a program that aims to meet the intended goals; the program theory and design seek primarily to answer the question: how and in what tools should the program be carried out? The answer to this question leads to imagining the instruments to utilize that can respond effectively and efficiently to the problem. In the context of Covid-19, the Maghreb countries joined most governments in the world in using a multitude of instruments to change the public behavior and enforce desired outcomes. Examples of these instruments are: Legislative measures in relation to lockdown, curfews, face mask wearing, etc. Media campaigns were also utilized to raise awareness about the danger of the pandemic and also to advise the audience about best practices to prevent infections such as hand washing, social distancing, correct ways for coughing, etc.

Program process: this domain of evaluation can also be described as "program monitoring" the program delivery keeps going. This domain of evaluation is related to the implementation and delivery of the program as well as the experiences of the recipients. In this regard, the evaluator seeks to answer the questions on how well the program runs and what impressions the recipients have about the services/actions administered to respond to the social problem. Applying the policy response against Covid-19 in the Maghreb countries, we can identify a divergence of program process due to various reasons pertaining to internal policy factors as well as external factors existing since pre-pandemic era. The divergence in program process emerges over time as the future of the global sanitary crisis is unpredictable.

Program impact: this domain of program evaluation addresses the effectiveness of the program. It asked whether the desired goals which were set in the program design are met. However, impact evaluation can be influenced by non-policy or program factors. For example, the quick success of Tunisia's policy against the first wave of Covid-19 may not be attributed to the program alone. The quick reopening in May 2020 may be due to low population of the country, compared to Algeria and Tunisia. Still, "the size of the recipient" factor, though not related to the program, helped speed up the process. Another important challenge with impact evaluation is the continuity of the crisis as well as uncertainty surrounding its future. This chapter tries, however, to measure the policy impact after three waves of the pandemic. Thus, based on epidemiological data, when the infection and death rates lower to the minimum levels, this is an indicator of policy effectiveness until the curve rises again, then a new program evaluation analysis is required. Besides, programs targeting socio-economic consequences are taken into account as parallel programs within the so called "crisis" policy.

Program efficiency: this domain deals with cost required or borne with the implementation of the program and its effects. Evaluator may conduct a cost-benefit analysis or cost-effectiveness analysis to weigh the economic impact of the program. Program efficiency is mostly concerned with money spent on the program. Therefore, it seeks to see if the program runs reasonably and efficiently without waste or excessive expenditure. Relating to the Covid-19 pandemic in the Maghreb countries, respective governments have used different funding strategies for countering the spread of the disease as well as mitigating its socio-economic impact. For example, Morocco and Tunisia relied on loans provided by foreign banking institutions, while Algeria adopted a monetary policy based on austerity and increase of production of oil and gas in spite of the fall of prices in the global market.

It is important to assert that the fulfillment of evaluation through the five domains presented above is embedded in the macroeconomic model of input-output of program and organization. In this respect, we have to identify the input, output and also outcome of a policy before we conduct an evaluation study. The input-output model in program or organization allows policy researchers and evaluators recognize the first five stages of policy cycle: agenda setting, policy formulation, policy adoption and then policy implementation. The fifth stage, which is evaluation, reviews the previous steps with the aim to improve, redesign or simply bring about knowledge about a policy issue. Figure 8.1 shows the process of evaluation and feedback in the general governance model, which is also relevant to public policy, among which anti-conid-19 policy.

The policy evaluation starts with objectives that are framed according to the public needs (in the case of anti-Covid-19 policy, the objectives would be to reduce cases of deaths and infections as well as mitigate the socio-economic consequences), then policymakers respond to those needs by

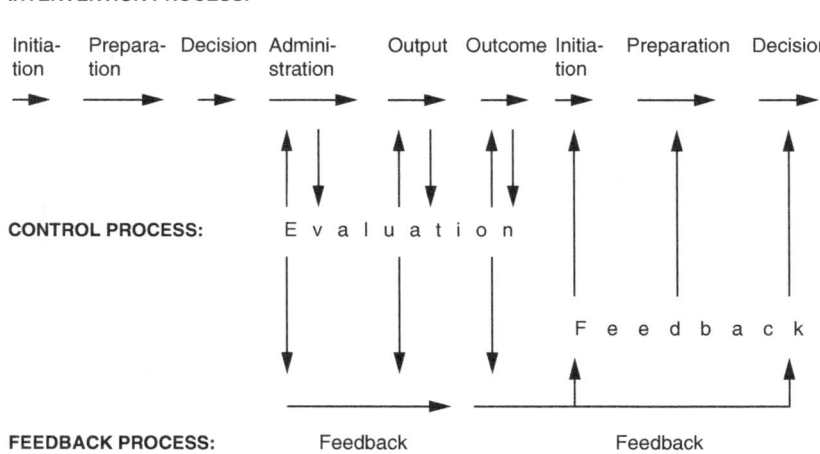

Figure 8.1 Evaluation of the general governance model

taking actions, represented in the figure as activities (in the case of anti-Covid-19 policy, inputs and activities can be merged together as policy instruments such as legislative measures, media campaigns, compensation on loss of job, etc.). The policy results are outputs in which an impact may or may not occur (in the case of anti-Covid-19 policy. Outputs are whether people respect the state of health emergency and related measures, including abiding by lockdown and mask wearing. Or whether all people affected receive compensation). Last but not least, depending on efficiency and effectiveness of the policy, final outcomes are the desired goal that were aimed to resolve the issue or responds to the needs (in case of anti-Covid-19 policy, the final outcomes are the status of infection and death rate, it could be as well the level of public satisfaction from social compensations due to loss of employment).

Putting the policy response against Covid-19 in comparative approach allows us to determine not only why a country/government chooses one or a set of policy instruments while another adopts a different one. Contemporary public policy scholars agree that comparing policies across socio-political entities can help us identify why a policy is successful and the other not (different policy outcomes). In other words, scholars in comparative public policy[3] "seek to explain why and under what conditions policy-makers agree on what policies."[4] Comparative public policy therefore can be used as a technique for determining the level of efficiency and effectiveness of a policy in different socio-political contexts.

As far as the case selection rationale is concerned, this chapter adopts the "method of difference,"[5] also known as "most similar systems design."[6] This method suggests that the cases compared (Morocco, Algeria and Tunisia) have similar social, cultural and historical characteristics, but the measures adopted against Covid-19 showed different policy inputs, outputs and outcomes as the findings of this research reveal. Therefore, the comparative approach and the method of difference help us to understand the factors behind existing variances in the policy against Covid-19 pandemic between the much homogeneous Maghreb states.

Epidemiological Responses in Morocco, Tunisia and Algeria

Epidemiological Situation

On February 25, 2020, Algeria reported its first case of severe acute respiratory syndrome coronavirus 2 (SARS-CoV-2), commonly known as Covid-19, from an Italian man who arrived on February 17, 2020. This was also the first confirmed case in the Maghreb, and the second in Africa.[7] On March 2, 2020, Morocco[8] and Tunisia[9] recorded their first case of Covid-19 from expatriates returning from Italy. Following the first confirmed cases, governments of the Maghreb countries introduced epidemiological measures to contain the virus and control its transmission. But, like the rest of the world, the virus kept spreading to other regions within each country.

Figure 8.1 presents different levels of Covid-19 infections in the three Maghreb countries. The daily infection lines went up together in parallel during the early days of the pandemic, until the end of March as Tunisia recovered quickly by mid-May, while infection rate in Morocco remained unstable throughout the first wave of Covid-19. The variance in daily Covid-19 cases reflects the effectiveness of measures adopted to reduce infection. However, during the second wave, a spike in infection rate was recorded in all the three countries, especially in Tunisia and Morocco as cases of Covid-19 reached 6,000 in the latter and 5,800 in the latter. The third wave that started by February 2021 also saw an increase of confirmed infections but less than the previous wave as vaccination campaigns reduced somehow the daily infection rates.

As soon as a dozen of cases were recorded in the Maghreb countries, the death rates simultaneously increased in Tunisia and Morocco, but significantly rose in Algeria until April 10 when the number of people dying from Covid-19 started to decline. Therefore, the parallel decrease of infections and deaths in Tunisia is due to several reasons, among which is the relatively better health system[10] which can smoothly serve the country's small population (11.6 million) compared to Algeria and Morocco (43 million and 36.5 million people respectively). Thus, the sanitary measures implemented by the Tunisian government succeeded to control the spread of the virus in only two months (March and April 2020).

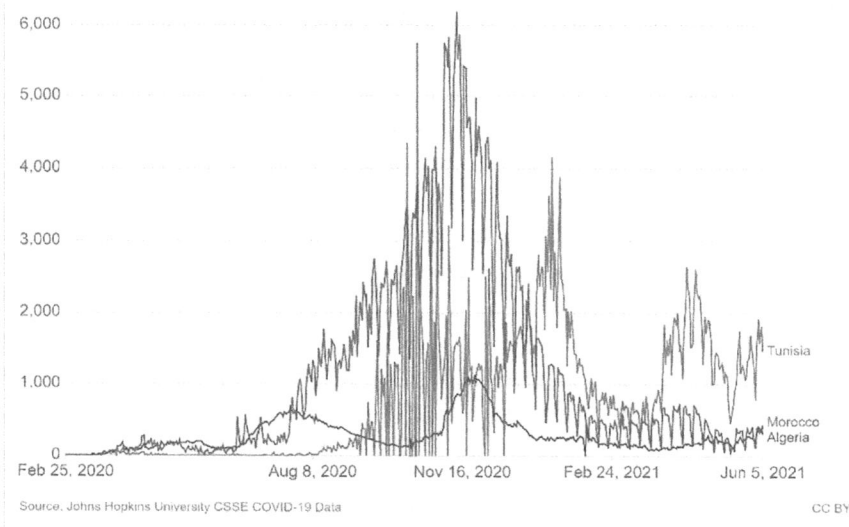

Source. Johns Hopkins University CSSE COVID-19 Data　　　　　　　　　　CC BY

Figure 8.2 Daily confirmed Covid-19 cases in Algeria, Morocco and Tunisia from February 25, 2020 to June 5, 2021

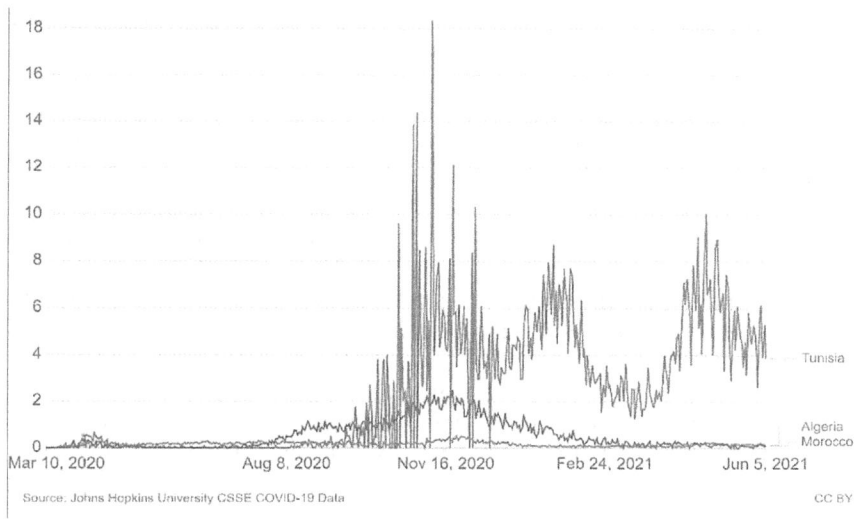

Figure 8.3 Daily deaths per million people in Algeria, Morocco and Tunisia due to Covid-19 from March 10, 2020 to June 5, 2021

It should be mentioned that high infection rates do not necessarily result in similar death rates as Figure 8.3 shows, compared to Figure 8.2. Morocco for example topped the Maghreb region in terms of number of cases during the second wave, but it came second behind Tunisia as the country with highest death rates. The variance between drop of deaths and increase of infections in Morocco could be explained by the early tracking of cases and massive testing of prospective patients, whereas in Algeria, the simultaneous increase of infections and deaths could be due to lack of public respect for the epidemiological measures such as face mask wearing, social distance or weak testing campaigns.

Covid-19 Testing

Polymerase chain reaction (PCR) tests are used not only as a tool in the fight against the epidemic but also as a source of data to calculate the number of cases, the proportion of positives or the incidence rate of the disease. World Health Organization even encourages mass testing to keep track of the spread of the virus which can help to contain it.[11] So, the more the number of PCR tests conducted, the clearer the situation with infection becomes. Therefore, the data regarding number of infections in daily manner can be misleading as to assume that in a country that conducts small testing campaigns towards suspicious and non-suspicious patients, it records smaller number of confirmed cases. However, if another country conducts more tests, and therefore records more cases of Covid-19, it shouldn't leave a conclusion that the lower number of Covid cases is due to its epidemiological policy compared to the second country with more tests and therefore higher rates of cases. That's why the number of tests administered each day is an important variable to take into account when determining if a policy outcome is effective or not.

When investigating the data on PCR testing in daily manner, there is unfortunately no information in this regard concerning Algeria and Tunisia since the beginning of the pandemic. It is until April 1, 2021 that Tunisia posts daily data on number of tests conducted each day. Morocco, on the other hand, started publishing daily updates on mass testing since the first case in March 2020.

Figure 8.4 clearly shows that the mass testing campaign conducted in Morocco and Tunisia could reveal the real cases of Covid-19 infection. Although the information on daily testing was not available in Tunisia before April 2, 2021, we can detect that Tunisia performed more tests than Morocco per capita in the first half of the year 2021. Thus, mass testing is an important part of the epidemiological policy to track and monitor the spread of the virus. On the other hand, absence of official data on testing in Algeria has caused speculations about the real numbers regarding confirmed cases of infection and number of deaths caused by the Covid-19 disease. Although Algerian ministry of health reported that over 2,500 tests were conducted daily by July 2020,[12] after a spike of cases of coronavirus

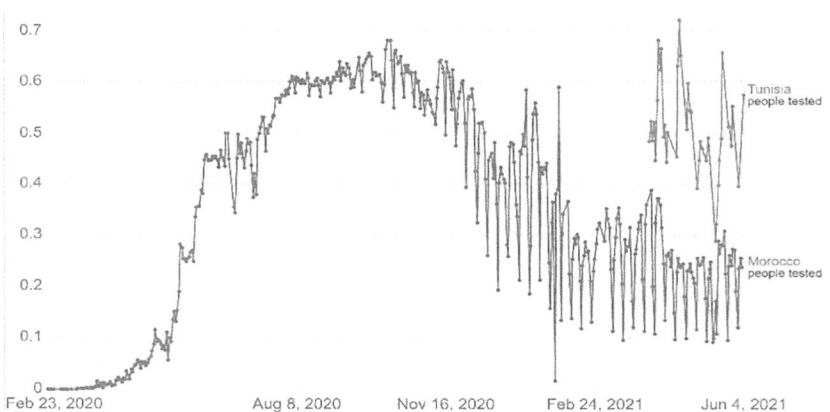

Figure 8.4 Daily COVID-19 tests per thousand people were administered in Morocco and Tunisia from February 23, 2020 to June 4, 2021

infection and deaths, exceeding the threshold of 1,000 by the end of October 2020, the situation could have raised the fear of Algerians for a potential mass infection higher than officially recorded. The high cost of tests available at the level of private clinics and laboratories had also increased the suffering of patients or suspected of being infected with the virus, which prevented many citizens from being diagnosed, especially with patients who had serious complications that could lead to health deterioration if the virus is present in their bodies.[13]

On this issue, local media reported that the majority of citizens, especially in Algiers, complained about the high price of the PCR examination, which amounts to 8,000 DA (about 50 Euros) per person in private clinics and radiology centers after being told by public hospitals that there weren't enough diagnostic devices which would meet all requests. The report noted that private clinics switched their policy from offering free tests in the early days of the pandemic into obliging people to pay for a diagnosis PCR test.[14]

In the height of the second wave of Covid-19 around October 2020, Tunisia was criticized for limiting number of tests administered daily to include only three categories of people: (1) every person suspected of having the disease and a carrier of its symptoms, (2) a health professional who had contact with a person infected with the Coronavirus or (3) contacts of positive cases of those who show symptoms only.[15] Head of the Examination Department at the Pasteur Institute in Tunis, Dr. Radhia revealed that the institutes had been exhausted by the number of Covid tests administered each day due to high demand and few logistical and human resources or even shortage of diagnosis kits required for conducting PCR tests.[16]

Morocco's testing capability could be described as sufficient thanks to decentralization of centers conducting PCR tests as well as the production of kits diagnosing the disease in a local Medical Biotechnology center[17] ensuring national self-sufficiency of such kits.[18] As of June 7, 2020, Morocco increased the number of tests and laboratories as more than 17,500 tests were being conducted every day in 24 laboratories across the country, while at the beginning of the pandemic, only three laboratories conducted about 2,000 tests every day. Mobile testing laboratories have also been gradually deployed across the country to achieve rapid testing.[19]

Government Responses to Covid-19 in Morocco, Tunisia and Algeria

The Case of Morocco

As soon as Morocco sensed the risk of COVID-19 entering into the country, the King of Morocco, Mohamed VI, held on March 17, 2020 a special meeting with key figures of the state, including Prime Minister Saad Edine Othmani, Interior Minister Abd Elouafi Laftit, Minister of Health Khaled

Ait Taleb, Army chief Abdel Fattah El waraq, Gendarmerie chief Mohamed Harmou, and the General Director of Moroccan security Abdellatif Hammouchi. This meeting outlined Morocco's response to the threat posed by COVID-19. Much of the attention and action was devoted to strengthening and reinforcing healthcare capacities in preparation for worse scenarios.

The government allocated 2 billion Dirhams (about 204 Million US$) to the Ministry of Health to be used in purchase of necessary medical equipment. As a result, the Minister of Economy and Finance declared that 406 intensive care beds were purchased bringing the total to 3,000, in addition to 580 normal beds as well as 410 respiratory ventilators. Most of this equipment came from China and South Korea.

Furthermore, the King ordered to activate military hospitals and to set up two military field hospitals with total capacity of 560. Another anti-Covid-19 field hospital with a capacity of 700 beds, including six intensive care beds was open after two weeks of construction. The field hospital is considered the largest of its kind in Africa (opened on April 20). By mid-April 2020, the Ministry of Industry produced over 500 Morocco made ventilators and more than 2 million units of facemasks daily by early June, securing therefore local needs for face masks. About 18.5 million units were shipped to 11 countries by June 8, announced Minister of Industry Hafid Alami.

On March 20, 2020, Morocco adopted the state of health emergency which gives extensive powers to the public authorities to take suitable measures aimed at containing the virus. The decision took place after a series of actions such as suspending sporting, artistic and cultural events and closing maritime, air and land borders, as well as mosques and schools. Other non-public spaces such as restaurants, barbershops and gyms were ordered to close. Right after the State of Health Emergency was adopted, more restrictive measures were ordered which included suspension of inter-city transportation and recruitment campaigns. Consequently, the authorities announced that everyone must stay at home except for buying food or medication or for work. In this regard, a document has to be carried by anyone going out, stating the purpose of his/her movement. Violation of orders within the framework of the State of Health Emergency will lead to jail between one and three months in addition to a fine ranging between 300 DH and 1,300 DH.

On April 6, 2020 as the number of COVID-19 soared for the third time, the government announced that facemasks have been mandatory for anyone leaving his/her place of residence. The new measure created public frustration because it came into force one day after it was announced, given shortage of facemasks in pharmacies and grocery stores. Within two weeks, textile companies managed to exclusively produce facemasks until they meet public needs. State of Health emergency had been extended every month since March 20, 2020. As of June 2021, at the time of conducting this research, the state of health emergency was in effect until July 10, 2021 when second relaxation measures were introduced, which involved waiving fully vaccinated persons from special licenses for movement during night curfew and inter-city travels. The latest easing measures also allowed mass gatherings up to a minimum number to be held in public and private places, as well as reopening of leisure and entertainment venues for a limited number of visitors.

The Case of Algeria

When faced with the increase of Covid-19 cases, the Algerian Government gradually took a series of general measures aimed at containing the spread of the virus since the first confirmed case on February 25, 2020. These measures were the subject of two main texts:

- *Executive Decree No. 20–69* of March 21, 2020 relating to measures to prevent and combat the spread of the Coronavirus (Covid-19), the purpose of which was to set social distancing measures intended to prevent and fight against the spread of COVID-19;
- *Executive Decree No. 20–70* of March 24, 2020 laying down additional measures to prevent and combat the spread of the Coronavirus (Covid-19) and which aims to set up devices for confinement, traffic restriction, 'supervision of trade and supply activities for citizens, distancing rules as well as the methods for public awareness.

These various measures were applicable throughout the national territory for a period which had been extended several times. Failure to comply with them is liable to lead to administrative sanctions (immediate withdrawal of administrative authorizations to carry out activities) and criminal sanctions without these being expressly defined. These restrictions were later followed by the closure of nurseries, schools, universities and training that had previously been operating.

Passenger transport activities were suspended for more than a year since February 2020 and this included: air services for the public transport of passengers on the domestic network; road transport on all routes (urban and suburban); passenger rail transport; guided transport (metro, tram, funiculars); transport by collective or individual taxi. This suspension does not however concern the transport of personnel which is the responsibility of the employers. In addition, the Minister of Transport and the Walis (regional governors) were responsible for organizing the transport of people necessary for the continuity of the public service and the maintenance of vital activities at the level of certain public services (health, safety, customs, etc.) as well as public institutions, administrations, economic entities and financial services.

Moreover, the government started to set up home containment operations for the population, either partially (that is to say during time slots defined by the public authorities) or completely. During periods of confinement, the movement of people was prohibited, except with exceptional authorization, for the following reasons: supply needs of authorized shops (food shops, pharmacies and shops relating to maintenance and hygiene).

The modalities for issuing these authorizations were defined by committees specially instituted at the level of the Wilayas. These commissions could also adapt the measures and take any other additional measures with regard to the specificities of the wilaya and the evolution of the Covid-19 situation. In addition, a compulsory measure was put in place, consisting of respecting a safety distance of at least 1 meter between two people; this measure applies to any administration and establishment open to the public and, as such, to all businesses and businesses not affected by the closure obligation.

With regard to retail businesses, most of them had to close with the exception of businesses, ensuring the supply of the population with food, cleaning and hygiene products, pharmaceutical and para-pharmaceuticals. But such businesses must conversely maintain their activities under restrictive human resources management.

The following institution and sectors of activity providing basic public services, particularly in terms of public hygiene, water supply, electricity and gas and telecommunications, were allowed to open postal, banking and insurance agencies; private health facilities, including medical offices, analytical laboratories and medical centers; fuel and energy product distribution companies.

On June 8, 2020, Algerian Prime Minister Abdelaziz Djerad unveiled the steps for lockdown relaxation under the guidelines of the health authorities. The first phase, which started on June 7, authorizes the resumption of 25 types of businesses and services, such as crafts, flower shops, hygiene products, cultural goods, the sale of takeaway food or the market cattle. As of June 14, other activities resumed, such as restaurants and taxi transportation.

As of June 2021, the Algerian government extended curfew from midnight until the next day at 4:00 a.m. in 19 wilayas (administrative regions) of the country from Saturday, May 22, as part of the ongoing efforts to control the spread of Covid-19.[20]

The Case of Tunisia

Following the formation of the new cabinet in Tunisia under Prime Minister Ilyass Fakhfakh, the Tunisian government adopted a set of measures aimed at curbing the spread of the Covid-19 pandemic in the country.

On March 12, air traffic was suspended with Italy, and schools and universities were ordered to close. The following day, the government announced further restrictions: cafes and restaurants would close starting from 4 p.m., collective prayers were banned, cancellation of conferences and cultural events, closure of maritime borders, suspension of flights with France, Spain, Egypt, United Kingdom and Germany, in addition to an obligation of 14 days quarantine for all people arriving in Tunisia. On March 18, full closure of land, maritime and air borders, banning of public gatherings was announced, imposing a curfew from 18:00 till 6:00. Obliging Tunisian expatriates abroad to self-isolate for 14 days with constant control. On March 22, the government announced total lockdown and ban on inter-city movement. On Thursday, April 16, a shipment of medical equipment was received from China. According to a statement from the Ministry of Health, the equipment was donated by China and the World Health Organization. These include screening tests, medical coveralls and gloves, and respirators to help fight the virus.[21]

On April 18, the President of the Republic Beji Caid Sebsi tasked a military medical team to set up a mobile military hospital in Kebili governorate to help with efforts to combat the coronavirus. Kebili was one of the governorates most affected by the spread of Covid-19 with 96 confirmed cases by then.[22] The country waited only until May 4th to announce the first phase of lockdown relaxation, however, not much long that Tunisian citizens enjoyed a "free" summer as the country entered into another nationwide lockdown in October, as the second wave of Covid-19 hit the country. The restrictions included ban on non-essential domestic travel, closure of cafes and restaurants, universities, schools, and places of worship. A curfew from 8:00 p.m. till 5:00 a.m. was also introduced.[23] These measures remained in force as of May 2021 as Tunisia battles the third wave of Covid-19 which Prime Minister Hichem Mechichi described as "the worst health crisis in its history."[24]

Covid-19 Vaccination in the Maghreb

In a continuous effort to battle the spread of Covid-19 and contain its mutations, it appeared for governments that preventive measures are not enough to force daily infections to drop to zero levels. Therefore, global pharmaceutical companies engaged in extensive clinical experiments to develop vaccines that are able to build immunity against the Covid-19 virus. By June 2021, World Health Organization granted emergency authorization to use five types of vaccines to be rolled out for the masses. These vaccines are officially labeled as Pviser/BioNTech, AstraZeneca-SK Bio, Janssen, Moderna and Sinopharm.[25] Although the distribution of vaccines worldwide stirred ethical debate regarding equality, the Maghreb countries pursued different strategies for the purchase and rolling of vaccine doses which also made an impact in the daily infections.

Based on the evolution of vaccination against Covid-19 in Figure 8.5, there is an evident variation in vaccination campaign between Algeria, Tunisia and Morocco. Morocco was the first country in the Maghreb to start mass vaccination against Covid-19 as King Mohamed VI kicked off the campaign on January 29, 2021.[26] Thus, Morocco can be seen as a leader in the frequency of vaccination during February and March with

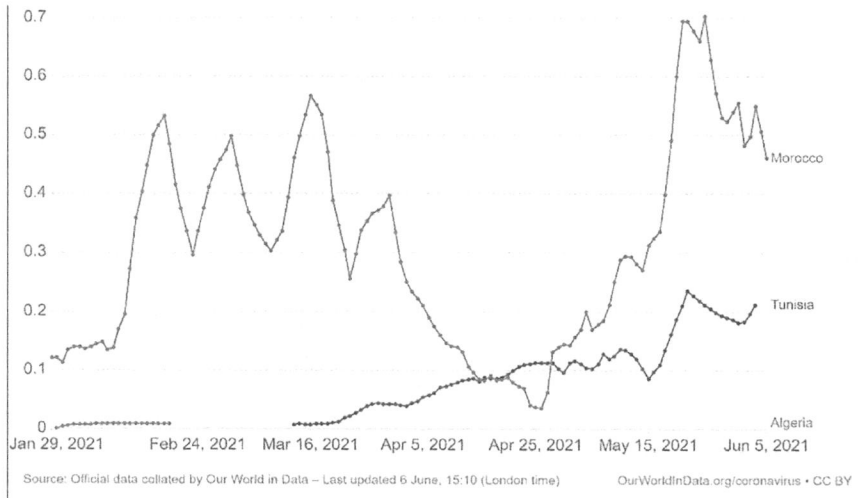

Figure 8.5 Daily Covid-19 vaccine doses per 100 people in Algeria, Tunisia and Morocco between January 29, 2021 and June 5, 2021

the number of people receiving their first dose recorded over 200,000 on March 16. Algeria launched its vaccination campaign on January 30 with a frequency of about 3,000 doses per day before the publishing of vaccination data halted on February 20. Tunisia started the vaccination campaign on March 13 through the COVID-19 Vaccines Global Access, abbreviated as COVAX, an initiative of the World Health Organization.

Vaccination Campaign in Morocco: Slow Pace after an Ambitious Start

The Moroccan strategy for vaccination against the emerging coronavirus envisages a large-scale vaccination campaign that is being implemented throughout the national territory. As of June 2021, Morocco used two types of vaccines: AstraZeneca and Sinopharm. The vaccine involved mobilization of 2,880 primary healthcare institutions, in addition to a large number of vaccination stations that are attached to them to develop vaccination activities through two patterns: (1) A persistent pattern: the population concerned moves to the vaccination station, mostly in urban and semi-urban areas. (2) Mobile mode: The vaccination teams attached to the station are transferred to the mobile vaccination points in rural areas according to a predetermined program, the number of which was determined at 7,000 points during the local planning. As of June 6, 2021, more than 9 million people aged 40 and above received the first dose of Covid-19 vaccine, while 5.8 million were fully vaccinated.[27]

By looking at the development of vaccination, Morocco recorded an increase in the frequency of administered doses in February and March, but soon the operation declined during April which can be due to two reasons: the first can be because of abstention by the public to take the vaccine during the holy month of Ramadan, as many fear the doses can affect their fasting, bearing in mind that similar shots such as insulin injection for diabetic persons break the fast, although doctors and Islamic clerics assert that the shots don't invalidate the fasting.[28] The second reason could be due to shortage of stock of doses, especially when the Indian Serum Institute that supplies the kingdom with AstraZeneca vaccines decided to delay shipments to Morocco, Saudi Arabia and Brazil due to high domestic demand as India topped the list as the world's most affected country by the third wave of Covid-19.[29] During the month of May, beginning of June 2021, Morocco increased the number of doses administered daily thanks to additional shipments provided within the framework of COVAX program.[30]

Vaccination Campaign in Tunisia: Late Vaccination, High Infection and Death Rates

On March 13, Tunisia officially kicked off its vaccination campaign against Covid-19 with the first shipment of Russian Sputnik V. People interested in the vaccine can have several options to book their appointments: either via a special website[31] dedicated for this purpose, by calling a free line, by sending an SMS to a designated number or simply by dialing with a code. As of June 1, 2021 more than 2.11 million people registered to get the first shot, although the category of people to be given priority for vaccination was still limited to teachers and staff in education sector, persons with chronic diseases and everyone above the age of 50.[32] The country aspired to vaccinate 50% of its population which accounts for only 5.2 million people. As of June 5, 2021, Tunisia authorized the use of five types of vaccines: SinoVac, Pviser/BioNTech, AstraZeneca, Sputnik-V and the single-dose Jansson of Johnson & Johnson.[33] It has administered a total of 1.05 million doses of vaccines, which is equal to 6% of vaccinated people receiving at least the first dose. Tunisia is set to receive 11 million and 700,000 doses of vaccines in 2021 through global and regional initiatives and through direct contracts with international laboratories.[34]

In spite of the late start, Tunisia's vaccination pace increased by May thanks to continuous shipments arriving in Tunis through COVAX program. However, it seems that the vaccination drive hasn't made much of an impact yet on the infection and death rates during April and May 2021, compared to Morocco and Algeria which recorded lowered rates per capita. The spokeswoman for the Ministry of Health, Nissaf Ben Alaya, admitted that the two weeks of May witnessed a very high level of alert at the national level and explained that the rate of emergence of positive cases carrying the Coronavirus exceeds 100 cases per 100,000 residents,[35] which puts Tunisia a high-risk country in spite of vaccination drive that keeps going at a growing speed. The reason for the high infection and death rates may be because of more tests than those conducted in Morocco and Algeria or could be due to ineffective measures tackling the spread of the virus as more than 100 variants were detected in Tunisia since April 28.[36] Others blame the public for not respecting the precautionary measures against the spread of the virus. Results of a survey conducted in February 2021 found that support for pandemic-related restrictions had fallen over from 61% in August 2020 to 46% in February 2021.[37] Moreover, only 35% of the respondents showed no intention to get the vaccine, which is the lowest rate among other people surveyed from the MENA region.[38]

Vaccination Campaign in Algeria: Lack of Inconsistence Data Stirs Questions

After it had officially launched its vaccination campaign on January 30, Algeria progressively increased its vaccination speed until it reached 3,748 doses per day as of February 19.[39] The data sharing on the vaccine development stopped later that date, which leaves Algerians uncertain how the campaign goes. The Minister of Health, Population and Hospital Reform, Abderrahmane Benbouzid, however, assured that the vaccination campaign against Covid-19 "would accelerate" in April, especially after the acquisition of further 920,000 doses from the Russian laboratory Sputnik and others provided through COVAX program.[40] For this purpose, a web portal was implemented to allow registration for people intending to get the vaccine under priority groups.[41] As of May 2021, the age group receiving the doses in Algeria is between 50 and 55 years using three types of vaccines: AstraZeneca, Sputnik-V and Sinopharm.[42]

In spite of the slow vaccination campaign, the coordinator of the Corona epidemic monitoring committee in Oran, Dr. Youssef Bukhari, said that the vaccination process was taking place according to the plan for which it was drawn up through 38 health institutions in the capital of the Algerian West, and that health authorities have begun to enable the age group between 50 and 55 years of vaccination to accelerate the pace of the vaccination campaign, in an effort to acquire the "herd immunity" that Algeria seeks to achieve after vaccinating more than 70% of the population.[43] Still, absence of official vaccination data in a daily basis could create speculations by the public about the progress of the campaign.

Policy Responses to Mitigate the Socio-Economic Consequences in the Maghreb

The Case of Morocco

In a bid to ease the effects caused by lockdown and closure of non-essential businesses, authorities announced they would double the currency trading band. On March 29, the Central Bank of Morocco announced a series of monetary measures to support access to credit for businesses and households by enhancing banks' refinancing capacity with the Central Bank. Also, a new fiscal law was adopted to allow Morocco to meet its foreign exchange needs, in particular, through the use of borrowing on the international market. As a result, Central bank of Morocco also received 3 billion US$ from the IMF as debt, to be paid in five years.

The fund that was launched by King Mohamed VI was valued as of April 28 at more than MAD 32 billion (approximately 3 billion USD), including 10 billion from the State's budget and 1.5 billion from the regions. This fund builds on the solidarity and contributions from the public sector, companies and private individuals who committed to financially support the country's efforts to contain the Virus and mitigate its consequences at both social and economic levels. Foreign development and financial institutions have also contributed to the fund such as the European Union (150 million Euros) and the French Development Agency (100 million Euros). The fund is monitored by a special committee within the ministry of economy and finance, known as "Yaqada" (meaning "watch"). As lockdown and closure measures were enforced, millions of employees in the private sector and businesses stopped working, including workers in the informal sector as well as freelancers and small business owners. The watch committee introduced a compensation scheme by subsidizing those people with a monthly stipend. The compensation method involves a digital platform for aid applicants (asking for their personal details: ID number, phone number, and evidence of their occupation). The amount for employees affiliated with the social security system would benefit from a 2,000 dirhams monthly allocation, while workers in the informal sector, starting with households benefiting from the medical assistance plan RAMED and which no longer have an income due to compulsory confinement, will receive 800 DH per month for households of two people or less; 1,000 DH per month for households of three to four people; 1,200 DH per month for households of more than four people.

The government also suspended payment of all social taxes until June 30. Banks also postponed loan payments for businesses and households who are facing financial difficulties. According to the Professional Group of Moroccan Banks, nearly 400,000 deferral requests have been processed with a rejection rate of 4%.

The Case of Algeria

The Bank of Algeria lowered its key interest rate from 3.25% to 3% and reduced the reserve requirement rate from 8% to 6%, in parallel with the easing of solvency and liquidity ratios. It also announced that banks and financial institutions could defer repayments of loan maturities or reschedule debt repayments of customers affected by economic problems caused by COVID-19. They can also grant additional loans to clients whose outstanding loans have been deferred or rescheduled. Business, consumption and personal tax payment deadlines have been postponed (except for large companies), and the recently introduced tax on retained earnings has been suspended. The recovery plan unveiled in August includes $20 billion in compensation for Algerians who lost their jobs as a result of the crisis, $11.5 billion in transfers to poor households and $16.5 billion in bonuses for workers in health.

In response to the social impact of Covid-19, authorities took several measures to provide immediate relief to households and to businesses. As of May 2020, there were 322,000 beneficiaries of the Allocation "forfaitaire de solidarité," which provided an allowance of 30,000 DZD per month to low-income job earners over the course of three months. In-kind support, consisting of food items and water, was also distributed to 600,000 households. Furthermore, the Ramadan solidarity grant was extended to 2.2 million households, with amounts raised from 6,000 DZD to 10,000 DZD.

The Case of Tunisia

The Central Bank of Tunisia lowered its main policy rate and invited banks to defer all loan repayments. The government also announced the creation of investment funds and sovereign guarantees for new loans. An emergency plan of 2.5 billion TND (about 2.2% of GDP) includes the postponement of social contributions and certain taxes, cash transfers and the free supply of electricity and running water for two months to vulnerable and low-income households (including the disabled and the homeless, retirees receiving a pension below a certain threshold, and the unemployed), housing for homeless people, the creation of a support fund of 300 million TND (US$103 million) for the benefit of SMEs and a package of liquidity easing measures for companies, to limit layoffs.

The economic recovery plan revealed in July 2020 maintains some of these measures, with regard to technical unemployment and state guaranteed loans, as well as the creation of a support fund for business retraining. A monitoring and support unit has been created for the benefit of companies hard hit by the coronavirus crisis. This unit strives to preserve jobs and safeguard the rights of employees. It also monitors the implementation of the measures taken. It is made up of representatives of the Ministries of Finance and Social Affairs, the Central Bank of Tunisia, the UTICA (employers 'organization), the UGTT (workers' union), the professional association of banks and financial institutions., and UTAP (Union of Agriculture and Fisheries). It is open to other ministries and organizations where appropriate.

The State released 3 billion dinars (about 1 billion euros) to finance an aid plan to support businesses and the poorest. However, these measures would be insufficient, especially for the poorest and workers in the informal sector who could not stop working overnight. In some cities, residents demonstrate against the authorities, despite the establishment of confinement, to denounce the lack of food.

Tunisia had also benefited from an EU grant of TND 800 million (US$276.5 million) to combat the crisis and its socio-economic consequences. Italy also offered a loan of EUR 50 million to the BCT in support of Tunisian companies and to mitigate the socio-economic impact of the crisis.

Discussion and Conclusions

The comparative approach provides a more robust explanation of policy effectiveness or success. Hence, management of the Covid-19 pandemic in the first wave in the three Maghreb countries reflects that collaborative, multi-actors-based policy is the key towards reducing infections, saving lives, and mitigating socio-economic impacts. By comparing three cases that share common social, economic, and cultural traits, it is the "consultation" based policy, among other factors, that determines success or failure of a policy. In this regard, the level of satisfaction by citizens towards their government's response was high in Tunisia and Morocco, compared to Algeria, which undergoes weekly protests against the regime. Figure 8.6 shows that

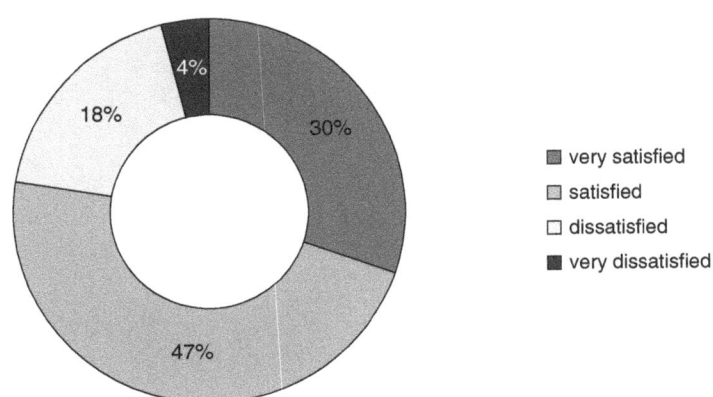

Figure 8.6 Degree of satisfaction with the measures taken by the government to respond to Covid-19 in Morocco

over 70% of Moroccan citizens were satisfied with the government measures against Covid-19. This data reflects citizen engagement with the government policy by abiding by the rules and restrictions such as lockdown and general health precautions.

Similarly, the Tunisian government gained public satisfaction with the measures taken in response to the spread of Covid-19. Figure 8.7 shows that 69% thought that the authorities did a good job introducing the precautionary measures to tackle the pandemic.

Regarding public satisfaction with the government's handling of the Covid-19 in Algeria, though there is no survey or poll conducted for the first wave of the pandemic, the Arab Barometer surprisingly indicated that the 65% of respondents rated positively the performance of their government in handling the covid-19 pandemic,[44] in spite of the political crisis and high death toll caused by Covid-19 until July 2020.

It is worth emphasizing that the Covid-19 second wave (September–January 2020) and third wave (February–April 2021) changed the government's strategies to manage increase of cases and tackle the socio-economic consequences. Public satisfaction also changed quite significantly when subsidies were limited or often cut. For example, Figure 8.8 demonstrates a sharp decrease of public satisfaction with government's policy towards Covid-19 in Tunisia from the first wave to the middle of the second wave.

The governments of Tunisia, Morocco and Algeria adopted a similar strategy to contain the spread of Covid-19 pandemic. The strategy included closure of borders, advice for hand sanitizers, social distancing, lockdown, etc. However, the difference in the policy lies in the structural as well as social relational aspects which produced different policy outcomes. This is relevant to the case of Morocco's strategy against Covid-19 during the first wave, which is based on a "collaborative" model involving the King,

Do you think that the Tunisian authorities did well in
the preventive measures against Covid-19 ?

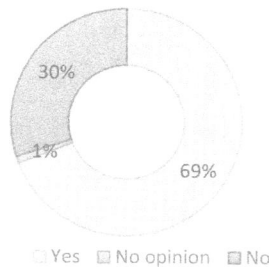

☐ Yes   ☐ No opinion   ☐ No

Figure 8.7 Degree of satisfaction with the measures taken by the government to respond to Covid-19 in Tunisia. Replicated from an Arabic-written pie chart

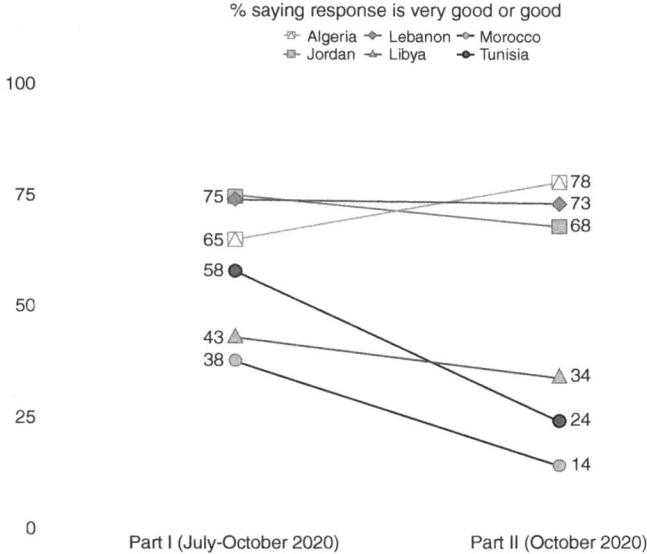

Figure 8.8 Changes in evaluations of governmental response to Covid-19 from July to October 2020

government and non-State actors who participated in the implementation of the sanitary measures and its socio-economic consequences, while, in Tunisia, which enjoys outstanding democratic institutions compared to Algeria and Morocco, it deploys its maximum human and financial resources allowing it reopen quickly in the first wave. On the other hand, Algeria's response to Covid-19 was met with public outrage against the regime which resulted in high death toll until the end of the first wave in July 2020. Nevertheless, the continuity of Covid-19 and uncertainty surrounding its future left all Maghreb countries to suffer from higher casualties during the second wave; meanwhile, public reaction and confidence in the governments lowered. The third wave of Covid-19 was marked with different vaccination campaigns carried out by Morocco, Tunisia and Algeria. During this period, the vaccination campaigns witnessed slow pace as dose supplies arrived in small quantities amid growing public disrespect of the precautionary practices and hesitation to take the vaccine.

Notes

1 Data retrieved from the John Hopkins University coronavirus portal: https://coronavirus.jhu.edu/map.html
2 Rossi, P. H., Lipsey, M. W., and Henry, G. T. (2018). *Evaluation: A systematic approach*. Sage Publications.

3 See for example: Lerner and Lasswell 1951; Windhoff-Héritier 1987; Howlett and Ramesh 2003.
4 Schmitt, S. (2012). Comparative approaches to the study of public policy-making. In *Routledge handbook of public policy* (pp. 47–61). Routledge.
5 Mill, J. S. (1875). A system of logic, ratiocinative and inductive: Being a connected view of the principles of evidence, and the methods of scientific investigation, Vol. 1.
6 Gerring, J. (2016). *Case study research: Principles and practices.* Cambridge University Press.
7 "Algerian Health Minister Confirms First COVID-19 Case | Africa Times. (February 25, 2020). https://africatimes.com/2020/02/25/algerian-health-minister-confirms-first-covid-19-case/
8 Morocco: Health Ministry Confirms First COVID-19 Case March 2 /Update 2. (n.d.). GardaWorld. Retrieved June 9, 2021, from https://www.garda.com/crisis24/news-alerts/319321/morocco-health-ministry-confirms-first-covid-19-case-march-2-update-2
9 Italian Returnee Confirmed Tunisia's First Coronavirus Case (March 2, 2020). *Punch Newspapers.* https://punchng.com/italian-returnee-confirmed-tunisias-first-coronavirus-case/
10 Abouzzohour, Y. (July 30, 2020). Tunisia may have beaten COVID-19, but challenges persist. *Brookings.* https://www.brookings.edu/opinions/tunisia-may-have-beaten-covid-19-but-challenges-persist/
11 WHO Publishes New Essential Diagnostics List and Urges Countries to Prioritize Investments in Testing. (n.d.). Retrieved June 9, 2021, from https://www.who.int/news/item/29-01-2021-who-publishes-new-essential-diagnostics-list-and-urges-countries-to-prioritize-investments-in-testing
12 Nassima, D. (n.d.-a). Covid-19: Les laboratoires privés autorisés à effectuer les tests PCR. Retrieved June 9, 2021, from https://www.aps.dz/sante-science-technologie/106866-covid-19-les-laboratoires-prives-autorises-a-effectuer-les-tests-pcr
13 "Algerian People's Daily - Expensive tests prevent citizens from early diagnosis," accessed June 9, 2021.
14 Ibid.
15 "COVID-19: Why does Tunisia continue to have limited tests?," accessed June 9, 2021.
16 Ibid.
17 MAScIR Develops a 100% Moroccan Diagnostic Kit for COVID-19 Testing. (n.d.). MAScIR. Retrieved June 9, 2021, from https://www.mascir.com/en/mascir-develops-a-100-moroccan-diagnostic-kit-for-covid-19-testing/
18 Morocco Produces New COVID-19 Test Kits. (June 16, 2020). https://www.eupoliticalreport.eu/morocco-produces-new-covid-19-test-kits/
19 Covid-19: Over 17,500 Tests Conducted Every Day in Morocco—Minister | MapNews. (n.d.). Retrieved June 9, 2021, from https://www.mapnews.ma/en/actualites/general/covid-19-over-17500-tests-conducted-every-day-morocco-minister
20 Covid-19: Reconduction des mesures de confinement dans 19 wilayas pour un mois à partir de samedi. (n.d.). Retrieved June 9, 2021, from https://www.aps.dz/algerie/121996-covid-19-reconduction-des-mesures-de-confinement-dans-19-wilayas-pour-un-mois-a-partir-de-samedi
21 Tests, respirateurs et équipements médicaux offerts par la Chine et l'OMS à la Tunisie. (n.d.). Retrieved June 9, 2021, from https://www.webdo.tn/2020/04/16/tests-respirateurs-et-equipements-medicaux-offerts-par-la-chine-et-loms-a-la-tunisie/#.YMEqf_kzZPZ
22 MKJ. (2020, April 28). Installation d'un hôpital militaire mobile à Kebili. Webdo. https://www.webdo.tn/2020/04/28/installation-dun-hopital-militaire-mobile-a-kebili/

23 Tunisia: Government Introduces New COVID-19 Restrictions and Extends Curfew Nationwide on October 29 /update 24. (n.d.). GardaWorld. Retrieved June 9, 2021, from https://www.garda.com/crisis24/news-alerts/394601/tunisia-government-introduces-new-covid-19-restrictions-and-extends-curfew-nation-wide-on-october-29-update-24
24 Tunisia Orders Lockdown Amid 'Worst' Ever Health Crisis | *Arab News.* (n.d.). Retrieved June 9, 2021, from https://www.arabnews.com/node/1855451/middle-east
25 WHO Lists Additional COVID-19 Vaccine for Emergency Use and Issues Interim Policy Recommendations. (n.d.). Retrieved June 9, 2021, from https://www.who.int/news/item/07-05-2021-who-lists-additional-covid-19-vaccine-for-emergency-use-and-issues-interim-policy-recommendations
26 ABC News (n.d.). Morocco's king kicks off country's virus vaccination drive. *ABC News.* Retrieved June 9, 2021, from https://abcnews.go.com/Health/wireStory/moroccos-king-kicks-off-countrys-virus-vaccination-drive-75543193
27 Data retrieved from the official vaccination website: https://www.liqahcorona.ma./ar
28 Ramadan: Experts Say COVID-19 Vaccines Do Not Invalidate Fast. (n.d.). Retrieved June 9, 2021, from https://www.moroccoworldnews.com/2021/03/336639/ramadan-experts-say-covid-19-vaccines-do-not-invalidate-fast
29 India's Serum to delay further vaccine shipments to Brazil, Morocco, Saudi—Source | Reuters. (n.d.). Retrieved June 9, 2021, from https://www.reuters.com/world/india/indias-serum-delay-further-vaccine-shipments-brazil-morocco-saudi-source-2021-03-21/
30 Covax Program: Morocco Receives 650,000 Doses of AstraZeneca Vaccine | The North Africa Post. (n.d.). Retrieved June 9, 2021, from https://northafricapost.com/49729-covax-program-morocco-receives-650000-doses-of-astrazeneca-vaccine.html
31 The website was down though, after being checked by the time of writing this research.
32 "At the Palais des Congres vaccination center: overcrowding and long waiting times," accessed June 9, 2021.
33 Autorisation de mise sur le marché tunisien du vaccin Janssen-Cilag. (n.d.). Retrieved June 9, 2021, from https://www.businessnews.com.tn/autorisation-de-mise-sur-le-mare-tunisien-du-vaccin-janssen-cilag, 520,107346,3
34 "One million and 700 thousand doses is Tunisia's share of Corona vaccines this year," Ultra Tunisia, accessed June 9, 2021.
35 "Ben Alaya: The alert level is very high, as we have exceeded 100 Corona injuries per 100,000 residents," Ultra Tunisia, accessed June 9, 2021.
36 Covid-19: Découverte de plus de 100 variants en Tunisie. (n.d.). Retrieved June 9, 2021, from https://www.mosaiquefm.net/fr/actualite-national-tunisie/889460/covid-19-decouverte-de-plus-de-100-variants-en-tunisie
37 Finding the Balance: Public Health and Social Measures in Tunisia, *Partnership for Evidence-Based Response to COVID-19* (third survey). February 2021. https://preventepidemics.org/wp content/uploads/2021/03/tunisia_en_20210316_2047.pdf
38 Ibid.
39 Algeria: The Latest Coronavirus Counts, Charts and Maps. (n.d.). Retrieved June 9, 2021, from https://graphics.reuters.com/world-coronavirus-tracker-and-maps/countries-and-territories/algeria/
40 Nassima, D. (n.d.-b). La campagne de vaccination anti-covid 19 s'accélèrera avril courant. Retrieved June 9, 2021, from https://www.aps.dz/sante-science-technologie/120017-la-campagne-de-vaccination-anti-covid-19-s-accelerera-avril-courant
41 The registration platform is http://vac-covid19.sante.gov.dz:9580/rdvac/menu_ins/, but it wasn't accessible at the time of writing this research in June 2021.

42 "Algeria news for Tuesday, May 18, 2021," Al Shorouk Online, May 18, 2021, https://www.echoroukonline.com/-2021ماي-18-الثلاثاء-ليوم-الجزائر-أخبار
43 Ibid.
44 Arabs' Evaluations of their Governments' Response to COVID-19 – Arab Barometer. (n.d.). Retrieved April 29, 2021, from https://www.arabbarometer. org/2020/12/arabs-evaluations-of-their-governments-response-to-covid-19/

References

ABC News (n.d.). Morocco's king kicks off country's virus vaccination drive. *ABC News*. Retrieved June 9, 2021, from https://abcnews.go.com/Health/wireStory/ moroccos-king-kicks-off-countrys-virus-vaccination-drive-75543193

Abouzzohour, Y. (2020, July 30). Tunisia may have beaten COVID-19, but challenges persist. *Brookings*. https://www.brookings.edu/opinions/tunisia-may-have-beaten-covid-19-but-challenges-persist/

Algeria: The Latest Coronavirus Counts, Charts and Maps. (n.d.). Retrieved June 9, 2021, from https://graphics.reuters.com/world-coronavirus-tracker-and-maps/ countries-and-territories/algeria/

Algerian Health Minister Confirms First COVID-19 Case | Africa Times. (2020, February 25). https://africatimes.com/2020/02/25/algerian-health-minister-confirms-first-covid-19-case/

Arabs' Evaluations of their Governments' Response to COVID-19 – Arab Barometer. (n.d.). Retrieved April 29, 2021, from https://www.arabbarometer.org/2020/12/ arabs-evaluations-of-their-governments-response-to-covid-19/

Autorisation de mise sur le marché tunisien du vaccin Janssen-Cilag. (n.d.). Retrieved June 9, 2021, from https://www.businessnews.com.tn/autorisation-de-mise-sur-le-mare-tunisien-du-vaccin-janssen-cilag, 520,107346,3

Covax Program: Morocco Receives 650,000 Doses of AstraZeneca Vaccine | The North Africa Post. (n.d.). Retrieved June 9, 2021, from https://northafricapost. com/49729-covax-program-morocco-receives-650000-doses-of-astrazeneca-vaccine.html

Covid-19: Découverte de plus de 100 variants en Tunisie. (n.d.). Retrieved June 9, 2021, from https://www.mosaiquefm.net/fr/actualite-national-tunisie/889460/ covid-19-decouverte-de-plus-de-100-variants-en-tunisie

Covid-19: Over 17,500 Tests Conducted Every Day in Morocco—Minister | MapNews. (n.d.). Retrieved June 9, 2021, from https://www.mapnews.ma/en/actualites/ general/covid-19-over-17500-tests-conducted-every-day-morocco-minister

Covid-19: Reconduction des mesures de confinement dans 19 wilayas pour un mois à partir de samedi. (n.d.). Retrieved June 9, 2021, from https://www.aps. dz/algerie/121996-covid-19-reconduction-des-mesures-de-confinement-dans-19-wilayas-pour-un-mois-a-partir-de-samedi

Gerring, J. (2016). *Case study research: Principles and practices*. Cambridge University Press, Cambridge, UK.

Howlett N., & Ramesh M. (2003). *Studying Public Policy: Policy Cycles and Policy Subsystems, Toronto*. Oxford University Press, Oxford, UK.

India's Serum to delay further vaccine shipments to Brazil, Morocco, Saudi—Source | Reuters. (n.d.). Retrieved June 9, 2021, from https://www.reuters.com/ world/india/indias-serum-delay-further-vaccine-shipments-brazil-morocco-saudi-source-2021-03-21/

Italian Returnee Confirmed Tunisia's First Coronavirus Case. (2020, March 2). *Punch Newspapers.* https://punchng.com/italian-returnee-confirmed-tunisias-first-coronavirus-case/

Lasswell, H. D., & Lerner D. (1951). The policy orientation. *Communication Researchers and Policy–Making*, 85–102.

MAScIR Develops a 100% Moroccan Diagnostic Kit for COVID-19 Testing. (n.d.). MAScIR. Retrieved June 9, 2021, from https://www.mascir.com/en/mascir-develops-a-100-moroccan-diagnostic-kit-for-covid-19-testing/

Mill, J. S. (1875). A system of logic, ratiocinative and inductive: Being a connected view of the principles of evidence, and the methods of scientific investigation, Vol. 1. Harper and Brothers, Chicago, US.

MKJ. (2020, April 28). Installation d'un hôpital militaire mobile à Kebili. Webdo. https://www.webdo.tn/2020/04/28/installation-dun-hopital-militaire-mobile-a-kebili/

Morocco: Health Ministry Confirms First COVID-19 Case March 2 /update 2. (n.d.). GardaWorld. Retrieved June 9, 2021, from https://www.garda.com/crisis24/news-alerts/319321/morocco-health-ministry-confirms-first-covid-19-case-march-2-update-2

Morocco Produces New COVID-19 Test Kits. (2020, June 16). https://www.eupoliticalreport.eu/morocco-produces-new-covid-19-test-kits/

Nassima, D. (n.d.-a). Covid-19: Les laboratoires privés autorisés à effectuer les tests PCR. Retrieved June 9, 2021, from https://www.aps.dz/sante-science-technologie/106866-covid-19-les-laboratoires-prives-autorises-a-effectuer-les-tests-pcr

Nassima, D. (n.d.-b). La campagne de vaccination anti-covid 19 s'accélèrera avril courant. Retrieved June 9, 2021, from https://www.aps.dz/sante-science-technologie/120017-la-campagne-de-vaccination-anti-covid-19-s-accelerera-avril-courant

Ramadan: Experts Say COVID-19 Vaccines Do Not Invalidate Fast. (n.d.). Retrieved June 9, 2021, from https://www.moroccoworldnews.com/2021/03/336639/ramadan-experts-say-covid-19-vaccines-do-not-invalidate-fast

Rossi, P. H., Lipsey, M. W., & Henry, G. T. (2018). *Evaluation: A systematic approach.* Sage Publications, New York, US.

Schmitt, S. (2012). Comparative approaches to the study of public policy-making. In *Routledge handbook of public policy* (pp. 47–61). Routledge, London, UK.

Tests, respirateurs et équipements médicaux offerts par la Chine et l'OMS à la Tunisie. (n.d.). Retrieved June 9, 2021, from https://www.webdo.tn/2020/04/16/tests-respirateurs-et-equipements-medicaux-offerts-par-la-chine-et-loms-a-la-tunisie/#.YMEqf_kzZPZ

Tunisia_en_20210316_2047.pdf. (n.d.). Retrieved June 9, 2021, from https://preventepidemics.org/wp-content/uploads/2021/03/tunisia_en_20210316_2047.pdf

Tunisia: Government Introduces New COVID-19 Restrictions and Extends Curfew Nationwide on October 29 /update 24. (n.d.). GardaWorld. Retrieved June 9, 2021, from https://www.garda.com/crisis24/news-alerts/394601/tunisia-government-introduces-new-covid-19-restrictions-and-extends-curfew-nationwide-on-october-29-update-24

Tunisia Orders Lockdown Amid 'Worst' Ever Health Crisis | *Arab News.* (n.d.). Retrieved June 9, 2021, from https://www.arabnews.com/node/1855451/middle-east

WHO Lists Additional COVID-19 Vaccine for Emergency Use and Issues Interim Policy Recommendations. (n.d.). Retrieved June 9, 2021, from https://www.who.int/news/item/07-05-2021-who-lists-additional-covid-19-vaccine-for-emergency-use-and-issues-interim-policy-recommendations

WHO Publishes New Essential Diagnostics List and Urges Countries to Prioritize Investments in Testing. (n.d.). Retrieved June 9, 2021, from https://www.who.int/news/item/29-01-2021-who-publishes-new-essential-diagnostics-list-and-urges-countries-to-prioritize-investments-in-testing

Windhoff-Héritier A. (1987). *Policy-Analyse*. Eine Einführung. Frankfurt/New York: Campus.

9 COVID-19 Policy Tracker

MENA Government Responses to the Crisis[1]

Andreas Rechkemmer, Ozcan Ozturk, Anis Ben Brik and Leslie A. Pal

Introduction

The tragedy of COVID-19 has coincided with a bonanza of comparative policy data. The tracking and mapping of *policy relevant statistics* is by now routine – interest rates, financial markets, unemployment, government expenditures and economic stimulus packages, trade balances, etc. – but the tracking of *public policy initiatives and measures* less so. And note that "tracking" and "mapping" are different from annual or periodic indices like the Worldwide Governance Indicators or the Corruption Perceptions Index (to name two of the most prominent). To "track" and "map" *policy* means to register government actions in real time, in the sequences in which they occur. Over longer periods of time, this can accumulate to a more or less comprehensive "profile" of sorts on the character, phenomenology, and tilt of a given government's policies in specific policy fields or areas. For example, tight budgets year-after-year are reasonable evidence of a contractionary fiscal policy stance (Raudla, Douglas, Randma-Liiv, & Savi, 2015). The accumulation over time of various policies in health, education, and social protection allows us to classify welfare states into various ideal types (Armingeon & Beyeler, 2004; Esping-Andersen, 1990; Schelkle, 2012). Tracking government actions on climate and the environment allows us to judge fidelity to the UNFCCC Paris Agreement (New Climate Institute, n.d.) or other multilateral environmental agreements (MEAs). COVID-19, similar to the 2008 financial crisis, provided a rare laboratory case of a single, global disastrous event that demanded rapid public health, economic, and social policy responses, as well as coordination at the regional and international level. Fortunately, events and hazards of this type and magnitude are rare, but they provide an unparalleled opportunity to track and map a rapid series of policy responses and measures that may vary by national circumstance and context, socio-cultural norms, institutional traditions, or political ideology. In this case, apart from the methodological enticement, there was of course genuine interest in comparing government policies to understand what worked best.

DOI: 10.4324/9781003266259-9

Coronavirus, Policy Trackers, and the PTGR

Policy trackers and governance indicators have grown in large numbers in the last few decades (Arndt & Oman, 2008; Buduru & Pal, 2010; Pal & Ireland, 2009), and by now number in the hundreds (Rotberg & Bhushan, 2015). Some of the most prominent include the Worldwide Governance Indicators (Kaufmann, Kraay, & Mastruzzi, 2010), the Corruption Perceptions Index and related measures (Mungiu-Pippidi, 2015; Mungiu-Pippidi & Dadašov, 2016; Mungiu-Pippidi & Johnston, 2017), and happiness indexes (Global Happiness Council, 2018; Helliwell, Layard, & Sachs, 2019; Stiglitz, Fitoussi, & Durand, 2018). This is a well-established field, but with virtually no examples tailored specifically for the MENA region.

The intense interest in government policy responses, actions and measures to the Sars-CoV-2 pandemic rapidly yielded an unusual number of new "policy trackers" and "dashboards" from different organizations and research entities, focusing on either specific policy fields or geo-political regions. This chapter focuses on one that was developed by the authors for the MENA region, the "COVID-19 Policy Tracker: MENA Government Responses to the Crisis" (hereinafter the PTGR). It comprises 12 Middle Eastern and North African countries: Algeria, Egypt, Jordan, Lebanon, Morocco, Tunisia, and the six Gulf Cooperation Council (GCC) states (Bahrain, Kuwait, Oman, Qatar, Saudi Arabia, the UAE) for the period of February 1, 2020 to January 31, 2021, tracking government policies and measures in public health, economic, and social policy. Methodological details and some of the most interesting findings are provided in this chapter. We present the data-gathering and analytical approaches, methods, and techniques, some of the key results and discuss observations and speculations on those results regarding the prevalence, character, and intensity of policy responses to the pandemic in the MENA region.

Table 9.1 presents a selection of COVID-19 related policy trackers. These are not primarily health status trackers (e.g., the number of cases, recoveries, and deaths linked to COVID-19), though in some cases (e.g., the Daily Clock) health data are presented along with records of policy responses, as well as policy recommendations. The most prominent health status related trackers are the Johns Hopkins University's Coronavirus Resource Centre ("COVID-19 Dashboard") (https://coronavirus.jhu.edu/map.html) and the WHO "Coronavirus Disease (COVID-19) Dashboard" (https://covid19.who.int/). A "policy tracker," however, self-evidently tracks government policy responses to the pandemic, and while these responses originally have been first and foremost in the public health field, they rapidly required economic (fiscal, monetary, and other), social (protections and other), and even international trade and mobility related policies. We discuss some of the methodological choices in constructing a "tracker" below, but at the moment, will simply note that trackers fall squarely within a solid tradition of governance and policy indicators (Bouckaert & Van Dooren, 2016; Bradley, 2015; Davis,

Fisher, Kingsbury, & Merry, 2012; Karabell, 2014; Maggetti & Gilardi, 2016; Merry, Davis, & Kingsbury, 2015; Pollitt, 2011; Rottenburg, Merry, Park, & Mugler, 2015). A recent development in the field has been the construction of various "indexes" that combine data and indicators into some more evaluative ranking or measure – Oxford University's Blavatnik School of Government "Coronavirus Government Response Tracker" for example tries to measure the "stringency" of policy responses to COVID-19.

Table 9.2 is a menu of the public health, economic, and social policy tools and instruments that have been available for or recommended to governments in dealing with and responding to the pandemic (there are some "micro-tools" that the OECD classifies as innovations, but they all fall within the categories listed in the Table). A few things stand out from this list and serve to remind us of the unusual nature of the pandemic as a policy challenge. The first point is the sheer scope of the responses that were required by governments. The first and immediate policy responses were in the public and human health field of course – e.g., mobilizing healthcare and hospital resources to deal with the sick, and ultimately the dying. That was almost immediately coupled with policy moves to ensure supplies of medical equipment, PPE, and staff. Testing regimes soon followed suit. Movement restrictions and closures (e.g., of borders, public places and businesses, and ultimately various forms of lockdowns) came close on the heels of the healthcare responses and were coupled almost immediately (as the nature of COVID-19 became more clear) with injunctions on mask wearing and physical distancing. More far-reaching and/or differentiated closures of, or access limitations to, public buildings, places, events and gatherings, individual and mass transportation infrastructure, and private businesses came afterwards and in many cases expanded to full lockdowns and stay-at-home mandates. But the scope and intensity of the pandemic disrupted economies worldwide and soon forced economic stimulus and other measures (as listed in the Table) as well as social protections through transfers of various kinds. All this is well known and documented, but it bears noting that to "track" and "map" policies in this specific case means tracking streams of actions across multiple and often (if not typically) disjointed policy fields – a challenging project.

A second point is that these policy measures were being announced almost daily, and in some cases, hourly. The pace eventually slowed after the first wave of infections, particularly in countries that soon succeeded in flattening the curve of cases. However, for the period from February to the end of 2020, most governments found themselves having to announce wave after wave of policy responses as the situation evolved and morphed in surprising and unanticipated directions, and the pandemic showed no sign of slowing down or abating (or if it did, only to come back in a second wave, third wave, and so on) mostly due to the emergence of ever new mutations and variants of the virus, inefficacy or lack of sustainability of government measures, and/or human-behavioral trends and patterns.

Table 9.1 COVID-19 policy trackers

Name	Sponsor	Link	Content (as of October 2020)
Country Policy Tracker	OECD	https://www.oecd.org/coronavirus/country-policy-tracker/	Fiscal and monetary, employment and social, and health. However, it also includes data on country responses in educational policy, science and innovation, tax policy, and supply of disinfectants. The scope of countries is different for each policy field, but the core consists of OECD member states and G20 non-OECD members.
OPSI COVID-19 Innovative Response Tracker	OECD	https://oecd-opsi.org/covid-response/	Innovative policy responses (submitted by governments). 434 entries, including information and practice sharing with public and/or internal; public service delivery under new circumstances; real-time data collection, sharing, and analysis; crowdsourcing responses; health and safety of responders; patient care; etc.
Social Protection Responses to COVID-19 Crisis Around the World Policy Responses to COVID-19	ILO	https://www.social-protection.org/gimi/ShowWiki.action?id=3417	206 countries and 1,496 measures, of which unemployment protection, income protection, housing, and special allowances account for over 50%. Health and food security are also included.
	IMF	https://www.imf.org/en/Topics/imf-and-covid19/Policy-Responses-to-COVID-19	Comprehensive and includes the key economic responses of 196 countries in fiscal policy (spending on health measures, support for households and firms, tax measures), monetary and macro-financial policy (interest rates, bond markets, liquidity provisions, bank credit, and lending facilities), and exchange rate and balance of payments (currency devaluations, foreign exchange marked interventions to mitigate volatility).
Coronavirus Government Response Tracker	Blavatnik School of Government, Oxford University	https://www.bsg.ox.ac.uk/research/research-projects/coronavirus-government-response-tracker	The Oxford tracker (OxCGRT) assembles 17 indicators for data from more than 160 countries in three areas: (1) containment and closure (e.g., school and workplace closing, public transport, international and domestic travel), (2) economic (e.g., income support and fiscal measures), and (3) health systems (e.g., testing, contact tracing, investment in COVID-19 vaccines). The data

COVID-19 Observatory in Latin America and the Caribbean	Economic Commission for Latin America and the Caribbean (UN	https://www.cepal.org/en/topics/covid-19	are assembled into four composite indexes on overall government response (which includes all the indicators and provides an index whether responses have become "stronger" or "weaker" over the pandemic), "stringency" (the strictness of lock-down measures), containment and health, and economic support.
			Monitors movement restrictions, health, economy, employment, social protection, education, and gender. It does so for the countries in the region, chronologically, and in terms of "actions" taken (with a narrative record of those actions for each country). "Social protection" includes cash transfers, food transfers/in-kind transfers, guarantee of basic services, and other social protection. The labor index include actions on labor protection (e.g., teleworking, paid work leave, paid sick leave, unemployment insurance, prevention of discrimination based on COVID-19, labor policies for low-wage, and/or informal workers), elective work leave, reduction of working hours, and prohibition of dismissal from work. For each of the seven tracking indicators, "story maps" are generated showing the number of "actions."
Daily Clock for COVID-19 in Arab Countries	Economic and Social Commission for Western Asia (UN)	https://www.unescwa.org/covid-19-prevalence-arab-countries	ESCWA draws on WHO and Ministries of Health data to provide a "daily clock" of the prevalence of COVID-19 in the Arab region, which includes (in declining order of number of cases): Saudi Arabia, Qatar, Egypt, the UAE, Kuwait, Oman, Iraq, Bahrain, Algeria, Morocco, Sudan, Djibouti, Somalia, Mauritania, Lebanon, Tunisia, Jordan, Yemen, Palestine, Libya, Comoros, and Syria.

(Continued)

Name	Sponsor	Link	Content (as of October 2020)
Coronavirus Disease (COVID-19) Dashboard	WHO	https://covid19.who.int/	Health impact data (confirmed cases, new cases, deaths) across the world, by country and by WHO region (Americas, Europe, Eastern Mediterranean, South-East Asia, Western Pacific, and Africa), similar Johns Hopkins University and the Coronatracker, though it presents the data in different ways. In addition, however, it provides "country guidance" and so is a source of global policy standards, benchmarks, and guidelines.
Policy Tracker of Government Responses (PTGR) to the COVID-19 crisis for the MENA region	College of Public Policy, Hamad Bin Khalifa University	https://www.menatracker.org	This site presents government responses to the coronavirus pandemic across the middle east and north Africa (MENA). The tacker assembles policy responses into three broad areas: (1) health (physical and social distancing/ workplaces; physical and social distancing/schools; physical and social distancing/mass gatherings; physical and social distancing/public spaces and transportation; movement measures; special protection measures/ persons at risk, vulnerable persons, and others; special protection measures/ health workers); (2) economic (fiscal responses; monetary responses; support to labor market; trade and supply chain; support to key sectors; support to other countries; reopening of the economy); and (3) social (access to education; care/healthcare/maternity care/childcare; children and family/maternity/parental leave; food and nutrition; housing/basic services; income/jobs protection/ unemployment benefits/injury benefits/sickness/benefits paid for loss of earning; pensions; special allowance/grant targeting vulnerable groups: women, refugees, disability).

A third feature, one that is not directly captured in the Table, is that even within a single policy field – building closures and entry restrictions, for example – there might be multiple, "micro-adjustments" that calibrate policy to address shifting conditions. These would include partial openings of religious establishments, adjusting the hours of opening for fitness centers and gyms, passing new regulations on social distancing in schools or entertainment complexes, revision to travel and visa regulations, the introduction or increase in fines for quarantine violations, revisions of lists of "low-risk countries," sending aid to specific countries, and so on. Most of the policy trackers listed in Table 9.1 took a selective approach – they would look at either gross changes in public health, economic, or social policy (usually captured through the announcements of the lead coordinating agency in each country) or as with the Blavatnk School, select several key indicators of policy shifts. Trying to take a full and complete snapshot of all policy responses, at all levels of government, in all sectors, and in both their macro- and micro-manifestations, is daunting.

The PTGR is similar methodologically to the ones listed in Table 9.1, but with several distinct features. The country selection comprised, as noted earlier, all six of the GCC states (Qatar, Kuwait, Bahrain, the UAE, Oman, Saudi Arabia) and a sample of six other Arab states (Morocco, Algeria, Tunisia, Egypt, Jordan, Lebanon) representing different sub-regions (Maghreb, North Africa, Levantine). Data collection focused on three main areas of government response to the pandemic: (1) public health interventions, (2) economic and finance interventions, and (3) social policy interventions. For each of these areas, further subcategories of policy measures and interventions were identified (to some extent paralleling those listed in Table 9.2): (a) public health: closings and movement restrictions; travel restrictions; contact tracing; isolation and quarantine; testing; case trajectories, etc.; (b) economic: fiscal and monetary measures; support for businesses and employees; production and supply chain; trade restrictions/incentives, etc.; and (c) social: education system; protection of populations, workers, families and vulnerable groups; religious observance; social services and welfare, etc. Researchers gathered qualitative and quantitative data on policy interventions in each area and subcategory for each country, by harvesting data from official inter-governmental bulletins and datasets (e.g., OECD, IMF, UN, WHO, ILO), official government bulletins, announcements, and websites (for each of the 12 countries), trusted news sources traced back to official sources, policy briefs and documents, and academic publications (using information in English, French, and Arabic). In addition, the project developed a custom-built search algorithm that mined significant additional data from official government social media and media accounts. Data were collected for the period February 1, 2020 through January 31, 2021, to amount to a day-to-day comprehensive tracker dataset comprising 12 countries, three main policy areas of pandemic response, and a total of 24 policy subcategories.

Table 9.2 Menu of policy responses to COVID-19

Public health measures

---

1 Personal measures for the populace: Frequent hand hygiene, social distancing, "respiratory etiquette," avoidance of groups, and gatherings
2 Physical and social distancing:
   a Workplace closures, except for essential services (pharmacies, grocery outlets). Encourage working from home as much as possible. This essentially was the "lockdown" that shuttered economies around the world.
   b School, college, university, and other educational institution closures, and/or partial openings.
   c Mass gatherings limited or prohibited, including sporting events and faith-based events (this affected the Islamic world particularly during the month of Ramadan from April 23 to May 23, 2020)
3 Movement measures: Closure of borders in some instances, restrictions in non-essential travel; internal restrictions for in-country movements.
4 Special protection measures:
   a Prisons and seniors' residences.
   b Migrants and refugees (especially in the Middle East and some African countries, where highly congested refugee camps made social distancing and even basic hygiene difficult).
   c Health workers: Organizing services and providing protective equipment for front-line workers.
5 Contact tracing measures: Manual tracking and more sophisticated use of IT and apps (some countries issued mandatory health and contact apps, such as Qatar's *Ehteraz*).

Economic policy measures (including monetary and fiscal)
1 Basic income support for workers (design features varied widely from single payments to top-ups and concessions on unemployment insurance claims).
2 Support for small business and specific sectors (e.g., airlines, tourism). This could be in the form of tax breaks or holidays, subsidies, buy-outs, etc.
3 Mortgage support.
4 Monetary policy (keeping interest rates low; bond market interventions).
5 Fiscal spending measures to reboot the economy.

Social policy measures (*Note: Some of these interventions overlap with public health and economic policy (protecting income) measures but were geared to protection of vulnerable groups specifically)*
1 Food transfers/in-kind transfers.
2 Paid work and sick leave.
3 Unemployment insurance.
4 Prevention of discrimination based on COVID-19.
5 Labor policies for low-wage and/or informal workers.

The methodology was deliberately agnostic. Unlike the Blavatnik index, which developed a metric of stringency, the PTGR approach was simply to track each measure taken by each of the 12 governments over the period under examination and thereby produce an interactive profile for each country as well as various comparative "maps." No single initiative or policy response is weighted more than others, and while the raw data will allow construction of indexes (the data are available on request), the project did not attempt to do this. However, by tracking each announcement across the three policy fields and their numerous subfields, it is possible to see patterns of response over time and also the relative balance within and across public health, economic, and social policy areas and, of course, compare all of these across the country sample.

Figure 9.1, for example, shows the acceleration of policy announce-ments from February through August 2020, climbing steeply in ten coun-tries compared here, and roughly at the same pace. The number of daily new policy announcements declined over the summer, but then picked up again in August. But the character of the announcements changed – in the February–March period, they were primarily about closures, lockdowns, and restrictions. In the August period, there was a gradual reopening and relaxation of measures.

Our comprehensive database of policy initiatives, measures, and inter-ventions was constructed in three phases. The first drew on existing policy trackers and datasets by UNESCWA, ILO, OECD, the IMF, and others (see Table 9.1). The second phase relied more heavily on official government websites and social media outlets, reports, media articles, and academic literature to provide a more finely grained and continuous reading of the stream of policy announcements coming from the respective governments (in three languages, English, Arabic, and French). The range of available and reliable sources varied by country – Saudi Arabia had the fewest, Leba-non the most, Qatar was somewhere in the middle. This reflected both a mix of the freedom of the press in each country and the intensity of international interest in different countries. In addition, we developed a search algorithm

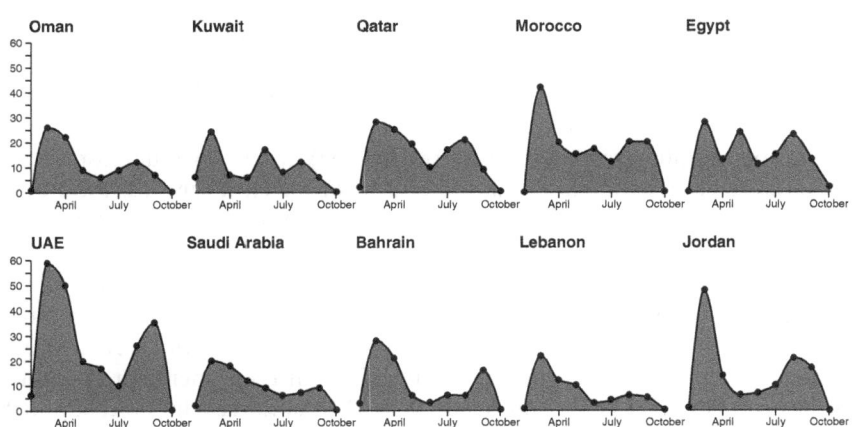

Figure 9.1 Monthly measures by country

to mine "hidden" announcements that official government accounts posted on websites and social media.

The third phase consisted of converting the manually generated data into a machine readable format in order to generate data visualizations and interactive graphics. Depending on the type of collection method involved, raw data can be a challenge to analyze and present. Automatic methods (through computers) and human-generated data often differ based on ease of collection, use, and visualization. In the initial data collection phase of the project, manual data collection was the main methodology used. The data were collected in Excel spreadsheet software with each sheet representing a separate country. The sheet includes three sections, public health, economic and social policy that were subdivided into a total of 24 sub-sections. As data were manually collected for each subcategory, they were entered in a new row in a cell under the specific subcategory with a date and description of the headline (e.g., July 1 – Up to 50% of staff can resume work from office starting July 1), along with a hyperlink attached that could be accessed by clicking on the cell leading to the original data source. The collected data were checked for mistakes and several quality check iterations were performed to ensure consistency in collection methods.

To better understand and visualize the findings, the data were converted to machine readable form with the help of Python programming language. A function was developed that could be called to easily convert any updated information collected manually. The function extracts the date, news headline, and the URL from each cell and transforms it into horizontal information that is machine readable and numerically usable (as can be seen in Figure 9.2). Once the data were readable in the programming language, various mathematical, analytical, and visualization codes were implemented to perform data analysis to find trends that can help identify trends of different policy measures used in each country.

Both fiscal and monetary economic measures were tracked. Fiscal measures included: (1) stimulus packages, (2) tax deferrals and/or exemptions, (3) wage subsidies, (4) deferment of debt obligations, and (5) support to SMEs. Monetary measures included: (1) policy rate adjustments, (2) exchange rate changes, and (3) liquidity injections into the financial system.

Nine social policy responses were tracked: (1) access to education (benefits in cash or in kind for the basic education of children), (2) food and nutrition (aimed at diminishing hunger or undernourishment), (3) income (wage subsidies, short-time work schemes, and other employment or income retention measures that could not be classified elsewhere), (4) social allowance (special allowances or grants to support different population groups against effects of COVID-19), (5) housing, (6) care services (access to essential services, including maternity care), (7) families (benefits provided to families to help meet costs and needs related to child-rearing and support of other dependents, (8) pensions, and (9) multiple functions (measures that

Economy	
Fiscal responses	**Monetary responses**
March 15 - A $1bn special fund (financed by the government and by tax deductible voluntary contributions from public and private entities) will	March 6 - As part of a gradual and orderly transition to a more flexible exchange rate regime, the authorities broadened the
March 16 - Businesses with less than 500 employees made temporarily idle and experiencing a reduction in turnover of more than 50	March 16 - Employees who become temporarily unemployed and are registered with the pension can put off debt payments
March 16 - All companies with an annual turnover of less than MAD 20 million can, if they wish, postpone their tax payment deadlines from	March 19 - The central bank reduced the policy rate by 25 bps to 2.0 percent.

Country	Category	SubCategory	Date	Policy	URL
Morocco	Economy	Fiscal responses	2020-03-15 00:00:00	A $1bn special fund (financed by the govern	http://www
Morocco	Economy	Fiscal responses	2020-03-16 00:00:00	Businesses with less than 500 employees ma	https://www
Morocco	Economy	Fiscal responses	2020-03-16 00:00:00	All companies with an annual turnover of les	https://www
Morocco	Economy	Monetary responses	2020-03-06 00:00:00	As part of a gradual and orderly transition to	https://www
Morocco	Economy	Monetary responses	2020-03-16 00:00:00	Employees who become temporarily unempl	https://www
Morocco	Economy	Monetary responses	2020-03-19 00:00:00	The central bank reduced the policy rate by 2	https://www

Figure 9.2 Human to machine readable conversion

concern several functions such as healthcare, access to education, children, and families).

The public health responses that were tracked followed the WHO taxonomy of the following recommended measures: (1) personal measures, (2) physical and social distancing in workplaces, schools, mass gatherings, public spaces, and public transportation, (3) movement measures, and (4) special protection measures for persons at risk, vulnerable and other persons, and health workers.

Results and Findings

Public Health Policy Measures

We tracked and mapped public health related policy responses, interventions, and measures across eight predefined categories: personal measures; physical and social distancing at workplaces, schools, mass gatherings, as well as public spaces and transportation (counting as four distinct categories); movement measures; and special protection measures for persons at risk, vulnerable persons and others as well as for health workers (counting as two distinct categories). This categorization followed that of the WHO's interim guidance documents released in May 2020 (World Health Organization, 2020). While taxonomies and categorizations of public health measures recommended to governments have varied to some extent, the one that we chose to apply in our tracker has been used consistently by the WHO and its pertinent committees. We rigorously applied our tracking methodology as outlined above and cleaned the data making sure that each tracked public health measure appeared only once in our dataset and in the category that fits the nature of the measure best. We only accounted for significant measures per WHO's taxonomy and guidance for the public health field and we cleaned our dataset for measures that were limited to a very local level.

In the tracking period (February 1, 2020 through January 31, 2021), we identified a total of 1,172 public health measures taken by national governments across our sample of 12 MENA countries, distributed across the following four main public health categories and as follows:

- personal measures (159)
- physical and social distancing at workplaces, schools, mass gatherings, public spaces, and transportation (522)
- movement measures (336)
- special protection measures for persons at risk, vulnerable persons and others, and health workers (155)

This means that the 12 countries together directed some 44.5% of their measures to physical and social distancing (including partial or full closures and lockdowns) and some 29% to movement measures (including curfews and the partial or full closure of air, land, and sea boarders as well as domestic travel). In other words, a stunning 73.5% of all measures (nearly three quarters) were about movement and gathering restrictions while only 13.5% emphasized personal measures (including hygiene and mask wearing) and only 13% consisted of special protections for vulnerable groups.

Comparing the 12 countries of our sample, the country-by-country breakdown of measures in the four main categories looks as follows:

Algeria: Out of 96 total measures, 16 were in the personal measures category, 37 in the physical and social distancing category, 29 in the movement measures category, and 14 in the special protections category.

Bahrain: Out of 75 total measures, 16 were in the personal measures category, 39 in the physical and social distancing category, 11 in the movement measures category, and 9 in the special protections category.

Egypt: Out of 100 total measures, 12 were in the personal measures category, 49 in the physical and social distancing category, 17 in the movement measures category, and 22 in the special protections category.

Jordan: Out of 118 total measures, 5 were in the personal measures category, 59 in the physical and social distancing category, 42 in the movement measures category, and 12 in the special protections category.

Kuwait: Out of 61 total measures, 8 were in the personal measures category, 27 in the physical and social distancing category, 19 in the movement measures category, and 7 in the special protections category.

Lebanon: Out of 65 total measures, 3 were in the personal measures category, 34 in the physical and social distancing category, 23 in the movement measures category, and 5 in the special protections category.

Morocco: Out of 116 total measures, 15 were in the personal measures category, 32 in the physical and social distancing category, 51 in the movement measures category, and 18 in the special protections category.

Oman: Out of 87 total measures, 11 were in the personal measures category, 37 in the physical and social distancing category, 31 in the movement measures category, and 8 in the special protections category.

Qatar: Out of 79 total measures, 12 were in the personal measures category, 40 in the physical and social distancing category, 12 in the movement measures category, and 15 in the special protections category.

Saudi Arabia: Out of 65 total measures, 14 were in the personal measures category, 34 in the physical and social distancing category, 14 in the movement measures category, and 3 in the special protections category.

Tunisia: Out of 89 total measures, 4 were in the personal measures category, 48 in the physical and social distancing category, 31 in the movement measures category, and 6 in the special protections category.

The UAE: Out of a stunning 221 total measures, 43 were in the personal measures category, 86 in the physical and social distancing category, 56 in the movement measures category, and 36 in the special protections category.

Obviously, the UAE took by far the most policy measures in the public health field. Since such measures are directly related to people, population size (along with density) matters in pandemic control. Normalized for population size, the UAE stands out even more, followed by Qatar, Bahrain, Oman, and Kuwait. It thus appears that the GCC countries were at the helm of public health measures in terms of the overall number, with the exception of Saudi Arabia, which may be explained by the sheer size of the country together with relative low population density.

Again, normalized for population size, among the Maghreb countries, Tunisia took more measures than Algeria and Morocco and those measures appear even more intense when the small country is compared to the vast territories of Morocco and even more so of Algeria. Egypt, on the other hand, with its 102 million by far the most populous country, appeared to have been least intense in taking public health measures, which is remarkable especially given that metro Cairo alone accounts for more than 20 million people.

Looking at the weight of measures taken within the four main categories across the sample, a few interesting insights emerged. While the distribution of measures across the four fields was statistically typical for Algeria and Egypt, Bahrain had a low amount of movement measures and Jordan had a low amount of personal measures. On the other hand, Jordan heavily emphasized social distancing and movement restrictions, being one of the most prolific countries in the entire region. Several countries (Kuwait, Lebanon,

Oman, Saudi Arabia, Tunisia) deemphasized special protection measures while Jordan, Lebanon, and Tunisia deemphasized personal measures. Morocco showed a high level of intensity in movement restrictions (with hard curfews and domestic travel restrictions in place especially during the first pandemic wave) whereas Saudi Arabia and Qatar displayed the least intense movement restrictions approach overall (Qatar especially in the air travel sector). The UAE led the field in all four main categories.

A more nuanced picture presents itself when public health measures are analyzed as a time series over the full 12-month period of our observation. For example, the UAE and Qatar issued a tight web of fairly stringent measures for physical and social distancing, including rigorous and sustained closures of businesses, hospitality, entertainment complexes, and education facilities early in the first wave while Bahrain, Kuwait, and Oman seemed reluctant to issue strict measures in spite of a spike in infections but acted on the physical and social distancing with a delay of several months. On the other hand, countries such as Morocco or the UAE reacted with very strict movement measures in the first wave but not so much during the second wave, although case numbers were higher then, presumably to avoid economic collaterals that occurred during the first wave. The full comparison of countries' measures in the various categories is possible using our dataset and visualizations on the open data web interface (Rechkemmer, Ozturk, Brik & Pal, 2020). It is also interesting to compare the results of our tracker with the University of Oxford's stringency index time series (Hale, Webster, Petherick, Phillips, and Kira 2020).

Economic Policy Measures

In the assessed time period, the region was impacted by two simultaneous shocks, the spread of COVID-19 and a sharp decline in oil prices. Though oil prices have been on the rise again since early 2021, oil exporting countries (OEC) lost significant revenue due to low oil prices in 2020. Oil importing countries (OIC), on the other hand, have witnessed a sharp drop in investments (mostly flowing from GCC countries), remittances, and tourism revenues.

To mitigate these combined effects, most governments in our sample have responded with several economic measures to protect households, the private sector, and financial markets. We tracked seven subcategories of such economic measures in the region: (1) fiscal responses, (2) monetary responses, (3) support to the labor market, (4) support to key sectors, (5) trade and supply chains, (6) support to/from other countries, and (7) reopening of the economy.

Fiscal responses in the MENA region have been broadly in line with other emerging economies. All countries introduced various levels of fiscal measures including stimulus packages, tax deferrals and tax exemptions, wage subsidies, and deferment of debt obligations. As shown in Figure 9.3, the size of the stimulus packages in the region ranges from 0% to 14% of real GDP. The average size for the region's stimulus package is 3.67%, which is significantly lower than the global average of 11%. The GCC subregion has a somewhat larger average (about 6%). The state of Qatar is noticeably an outlier with 14% in the size of its fiscal response. Although some measures adopted in 2020 have expired, with the waves of new variants, most fiscal responses (e.g. tax relief measures) have been extended and some new supports have been introduced (e.g., cash transfers, supports to SMEs, and vulnerable households).

MENA's central banks used conventional monetary policy levers such as cutting policy rates, exchange rate adjustments, and provision of liquidity into the financial system. The size of liquidity injections ranges from 0% to 29% of GDP. The average liquidity injection in the region is 9.7% while the global average is 15% of GDP. Bahrain has the highest rate with 29% followed by Oman (26%) and Qatar (9.3%). Although policy rates remained low in 2020, many countries have begun to tighten monetary responses because of inflationary effects. Some measures introduced in 2020 have expired while others (credit guarantees, repayment deferrals) have been extended. This monetary financing has caused rising inflation in the region and globally.

Regarding trade restricting and supply chain policies, responses during the Covid-19 pandemic were expected to be different from previous crises. During the financial crisis in 2007–2008, world food prices spiked due to low global stocks, high oil prices, and the adoption of strict trade restricting policies. In 2010–2011, food prices were high again caused by low production because of severe weather conditions. The Covid-19 pandemic is different

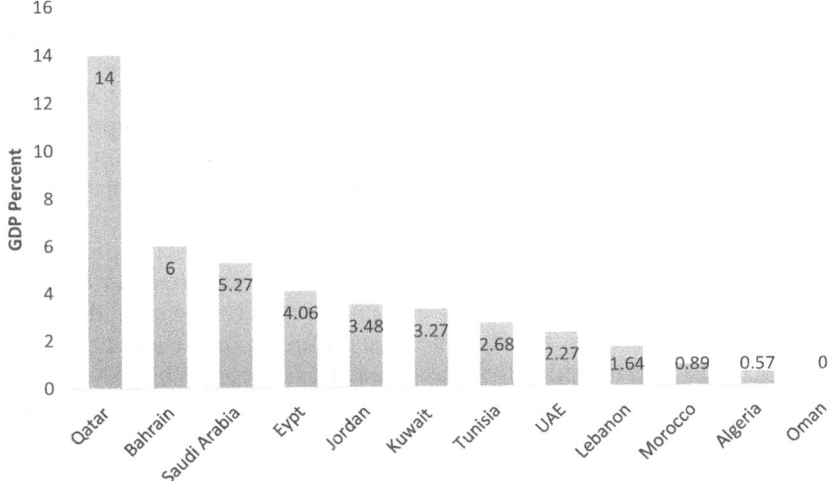

Figure 9.3 Stimulus packages in response to COVID-19

in that the production and stock level of most food commodities globally have been at all-time highs since 2015 and the prices of most staple foods have been stable since then until 2020 (then shot up in 2021). Empty shelves seen in many countries during the first wave of the pandemic were mostly the result of panic buying behaviors and/or local supply chain issues, not global supply issues. Hence, trade restricting policies should not have been a response to fight the pandemic. However, what was expected did not happen. Many countries around the world and in the MENA region adopted export restricting measures for exports of several products, including food, medical, and hygiene items. Morocco, Egypt, Saudi Arabia, Bahrain, and Oman adopted two export restricting measures each, while Jordan, Algeria, Lebanon, Kuwait, and the UAE adopted one each. Tunisia and Qatar imposed none. The high export bans only exacerbated the social and economic impacts of the pandemic. Although these restrictions were temporary, they played a role in high food inflation along with other reasons such as high input (energy) prices and monetary financing.

With regard to support to/from other countries, some countries (Qatar, the UAE, Bahrain, Oman, Kuwait, Saudi Arabia, Morocco, Egypt) sent aid to other countries in the region and beyond, to humanitarian organizations (e.g., the Red Cresent Movement) and to other international organizations such as UNICEF and WHO. Aid mostly included medical equipment, hygiene items, and vaccines in rare cases. On the other hand, some countries (Tunisia, Algeria, Jordan, Lebanon) received donations from countries in the region and the world and from international organizations such as IMF and WHO.

Social Policy Measures

Unprecedented precautionary social policy measures were applied to mitigate the virus's impact in the MENA region. A total of 269 measures were adopted. Access to education measures in the form of benefits in cash or in kind provided for children's basic education is the most common measure used by governments in the region (77 measures) followed by income/jobs protection and unemployment measures (43 measures) in the form of wage subsidies, short-time work schemes, and other employment or income retention measures that concern the labor market and benefits provided to a protected person arising from the loss of gainful employment (43 measures) and special social allowance/grant measures in the form of allowances and/or grants aimed to support vulnerable groups against the consequences of COVID-19 (43 measures). Other measures adopted by governments in the region included (i) food and nutrition (35 measures) in the form of benefits provided in order to ensure food security and adequate nutrition within households (these benefits are aimed specifically at significantly reducing or diminishing hunger, undernourishment due to food deprivation, malnutrition, vulnerability, and resilience); (ii) housing and basic services (19 measures) in the form of benefits provided in order to directly help a household meet the costs of housing and basic services; (iii) children and family measures (16 measures), in the form of benefits to help meet costs and needs related to child-rearing and the support of other dependents, income replacement for income loss from inability to work before and after child-birth or in connection with the adoption of a child, and parental benefits in case of interruption of work for child care responsibilities; (iv) pensions (seven measures) covering benefits paid to retired persons, survivor or persons with disabilities; and (v) measures that concern several functions mentioned above (29 measures) (see Figure 9.4).

The composition of social policy measures varies by country and subregion. The Gulf region has the largest share of social policy measures (55% of all measures), followed by North African countries (31% of all measures), and finally the Levant region (14%) (see Figure 9.5).

The UAE leads on social policy measures (15% of all measures) followed by Kuwait (13%), Bahrain (10%), and Jordan (10%). Lebanon, Oman, and Qatar have the lowest share of social policy responses (4%, 4%, and 5% of all measures, respectively) (see Figure 9.6).

While social policy responses in the UAE mostly revolved around access to education (17 measures), these claim large shares also in Kuwait (11 measures) and Bahrain (11 measures). Algeria and Morocco had the largest share of children and family measures (3 measures), while Kuwait leads on food and nutrition measures (9 measures) and Tunisia leads on special social allowances and grants (10 measures) (see Figure 9.7).

The timing of social policy responses is crucial. Waiting too long may lead to severe financial hardship in addition to the spread spiraling out of

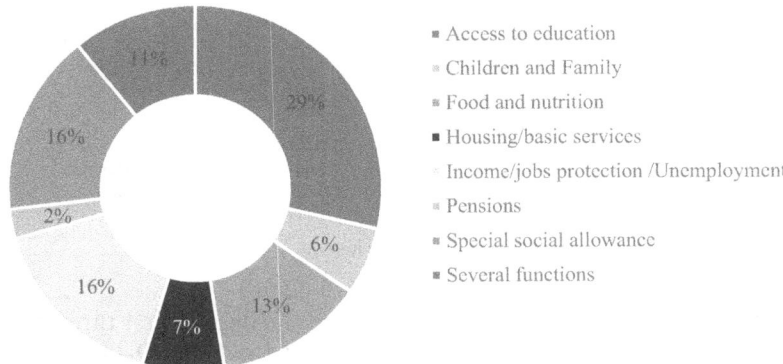

Figure 9.4 Social policy responses by category

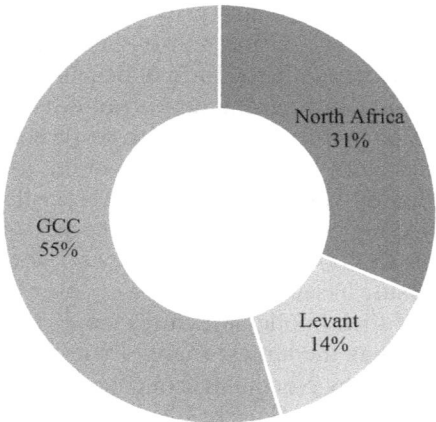

Figure 9.5 Social policy responses by subregion

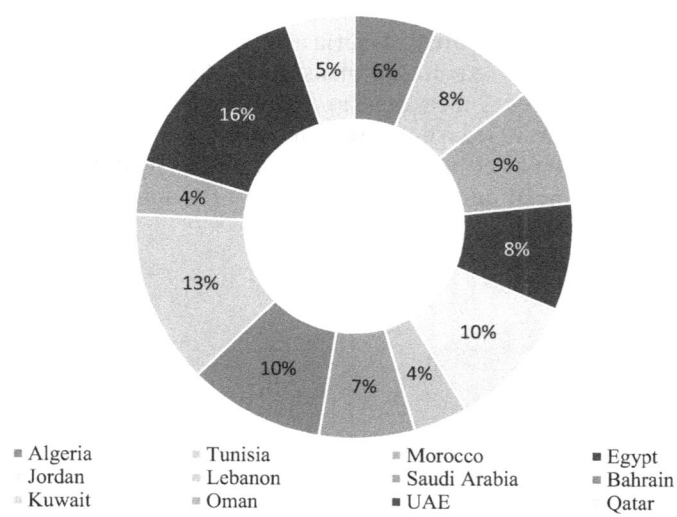

- Algeria   ▪ Tunisia   ▪ Morocco   ▪ Egypt
  Jordan   ▪ Lebanon   ▪ Saudi Arabia   ▪ Bahrain
  ▪ Kuwait   ▪ Oman   ▪ UAE   Qatar

Figure 9.6 Social policy responses by countries

control. Over 60% of measures were adopted during the first three months after the World Health Organization declared the COVID-19 outbreak a pandemic on March 11, 2020. 24% of social policy measures were adopted within the first month; 30% were adopted during the second month; and 7% of measures were adopted in the third month following the WHO announcement (see Figure 9.8).

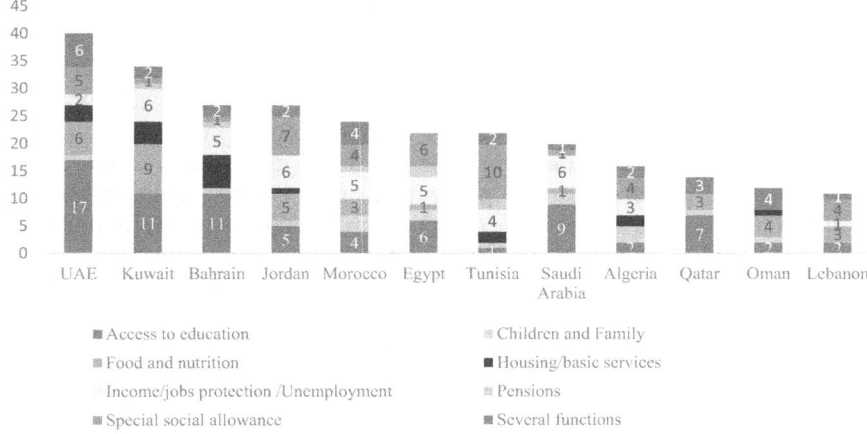

Figure 9.7 Social policy responses by categories by countries

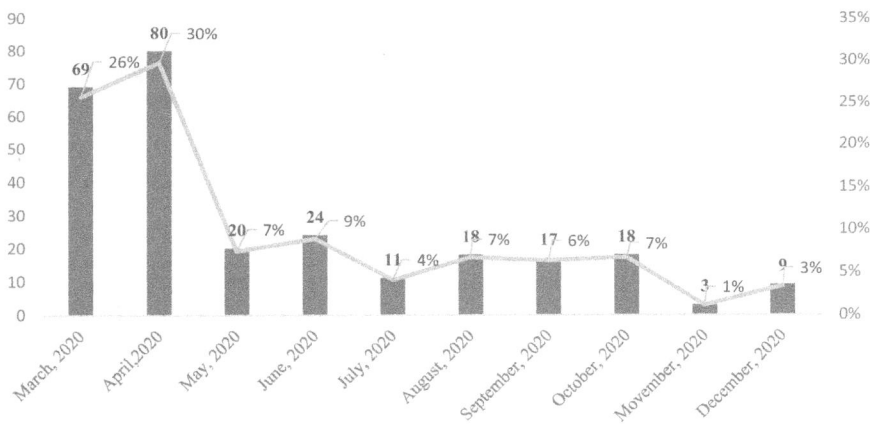

Figure 9.8 Trends in number of social policy measures, March–December 2020

It's worth pointing out that over 70% of social policy measures in five countries – Jordan, Tunisia, Oman, Lebanon, and the UAE – were adopted during the first three months following the WHO declaration of the COVID-19 outbreak a pandemic. While Tunisia and Jordan adopted nearly 90% of social policy measures during the first wave of the pandemic, Kuwait, Saudi Arabia, and Egypt adopted 26%, 40%, and 50% of measures, respectively, during the first wave. This means that many suffered financial hardship during the first wave period in these countries.

Overall, the majority of countries initiated social policy responses before the arrival of the peak number of daily new cases and governments' responses were upgraded after the WHO declared COVID-19 a pandemic. This indicates that the announcement of a pandemic triggered countries to act more aggressively against COVID-19. Moreover, the majority of countries had relatively shorter time spans of initiation, and the interval between initiation and upgrading to a high level was short. The interval from the first reported case to the time of highest response level reflects the agility of a government's response – depicting how quickly a government adopts comprehensive and aggressive social policy measures. Upgrading the response level to a high level in a short time can potentially prevent collateral damage from a pandemic. However, these responses varied across countries.

Our results identified six trajectories of social policy responses based on when the first response was initiated. First, some countries (e.g., Bahrain, Qatar, the UAE, and Algeria) started responses and upgraded to a high response level in a short time interval and kept a low or moderate response level for a longer period (see Figure 9.9).

Second, some countries started with a high response level in a short interval and kept a low or moderate response level for a short period, such as Lebanon, Jordan, Morocco, and Oman. The high peak of daily incidence in these countries came later than in countries where the first pattern was found. How homogeneous countries have been in the timing of the adoption of measures suggests that these countries were mimicking each other to respond to the COVID-19 pandemic and supports the claim that neighboring countries, those who share a border, those who share a religion and norms system, or

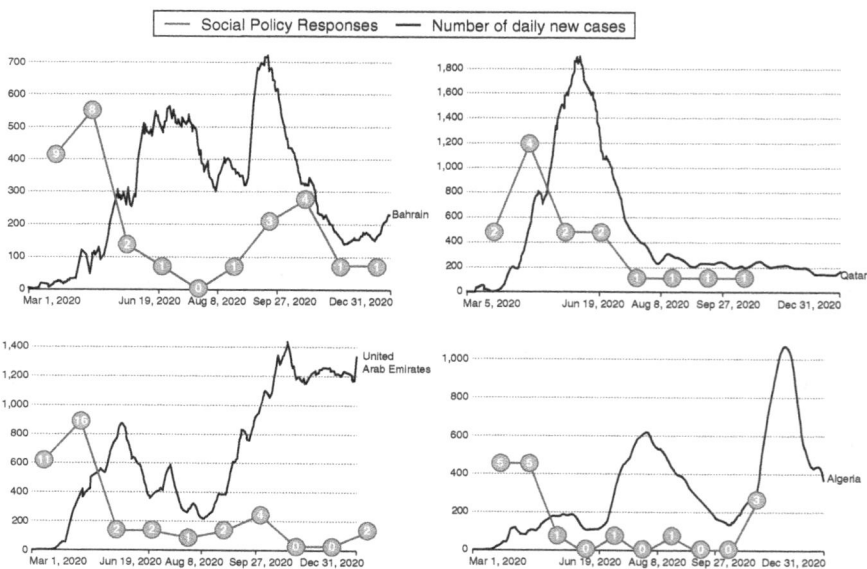

Figure 9.9 First trajectory of social policy responses and number of daily new cases in Bahrain, Qatar, the UAE, and Algeria, March–December 2020

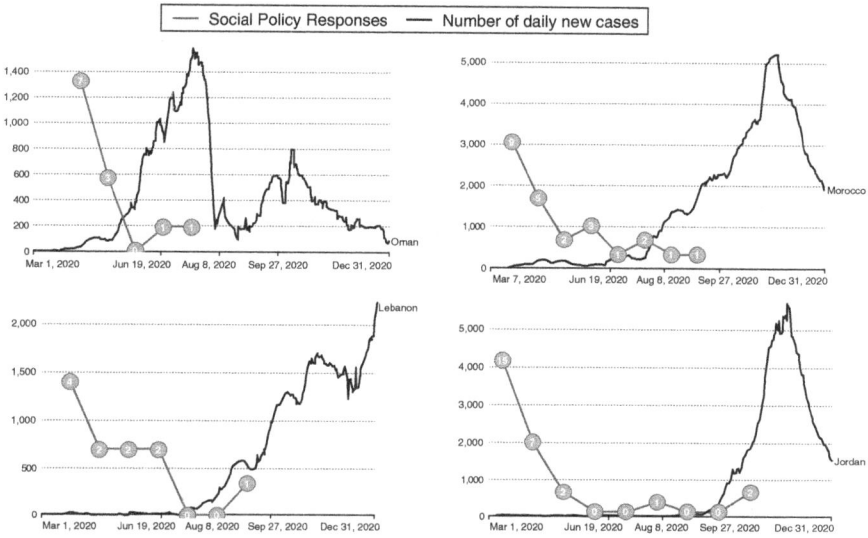

Figure 9.10 Second trajectory of social policy responses and number of daily new cases in Oman, Morocco, Lebanon, and Jordan, March–December 2020

those who have intense relations and share an interdependence, have often been shown to look to each other for adoption cues (Brinks and Coppedge, 2006; Leeson and Dean, 2009; Sebhatu et al., 2020) (see Figure 9.10).

Third, unlike countries in the second pattern, some countries like Kuwait took a long time before reaching a high response level three months after the WHO declared COVID-19 a pandemic). Kuwait upgraded to a high-level response in a stepwise fashion with a mixed scale and kept a low or moderate response for a longer period. The high-level response was associated with the peak number of daily new cases (see Figure 9.11).

Fourth, Tunisia started responses and upgraded to a high response level in a short time interval (six months before the peak number of daily new cases) and kept a low response for very short period (four months before the peak number of daily new cases) (see Figure 9.12).

Fifth, Egypt started with a high response level in a short interval (three months before the peak number of daily new cases) and kept a very low response at peak and upgraded in three steps with a mixed scale. The Egyptian government's responses were upgraded with further spread of COVID-19 in December 2020 (see Figure 9.13).

Sixth, although Saudi Arabia adopted at first social policy schemes and upgraded responses to a high level in a short time interval (three months before the peak number of daily new cases), the second upgrade of responses started at a later stage (two to three months after the peak number of daily new cases) (see Figure 9.14).

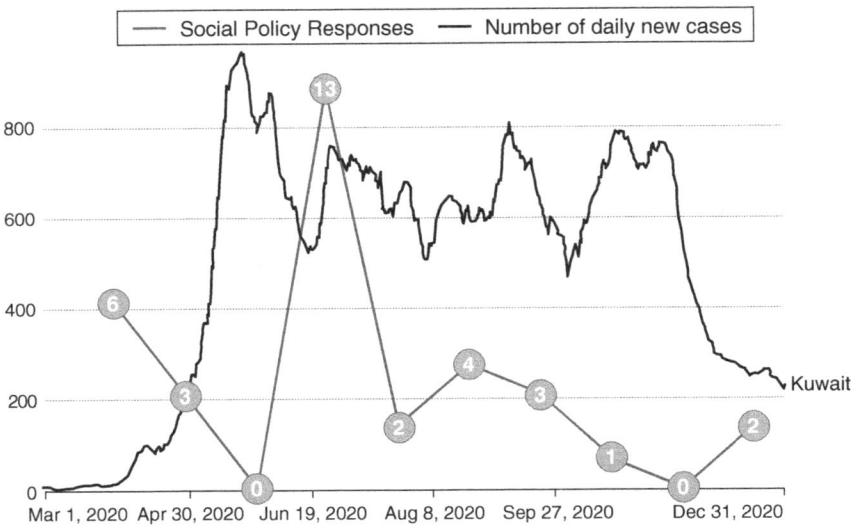

Figure 9.11 Third trajectory of social policy responses and number of daily new cases in Kuwait, March–December 2020

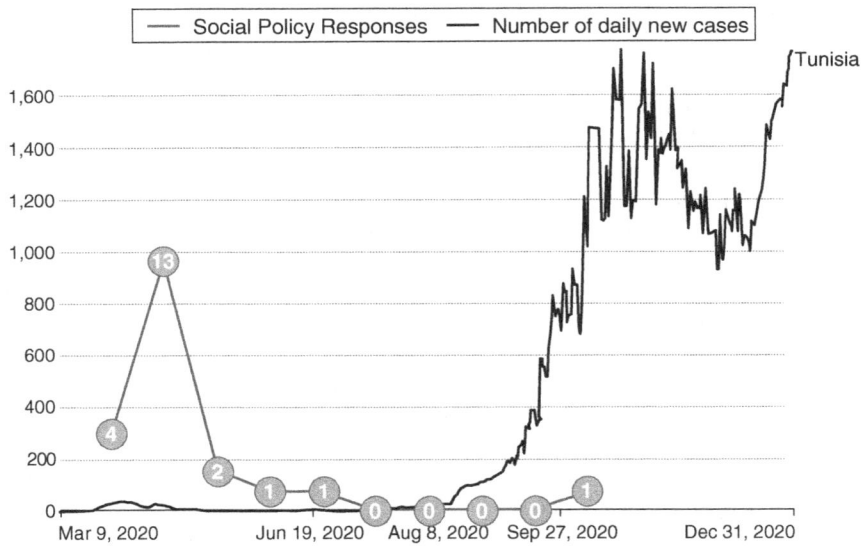

Figure 9.12 Fourth trajectory of social policy responses and number of daily new cases in Tunisia, March–December 2020

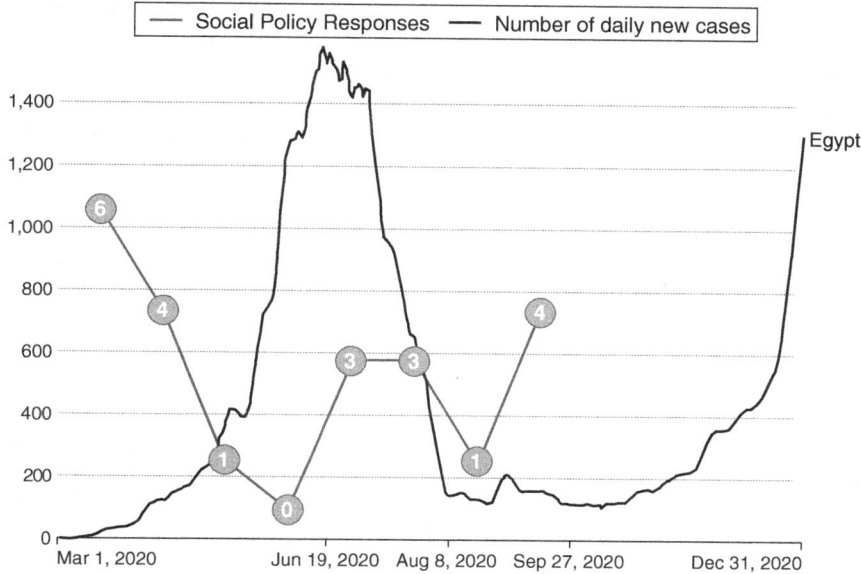

Figure 9.13 Fifth trajectory of social policy responses and number of daily new cases in Egypt, March–December 2020

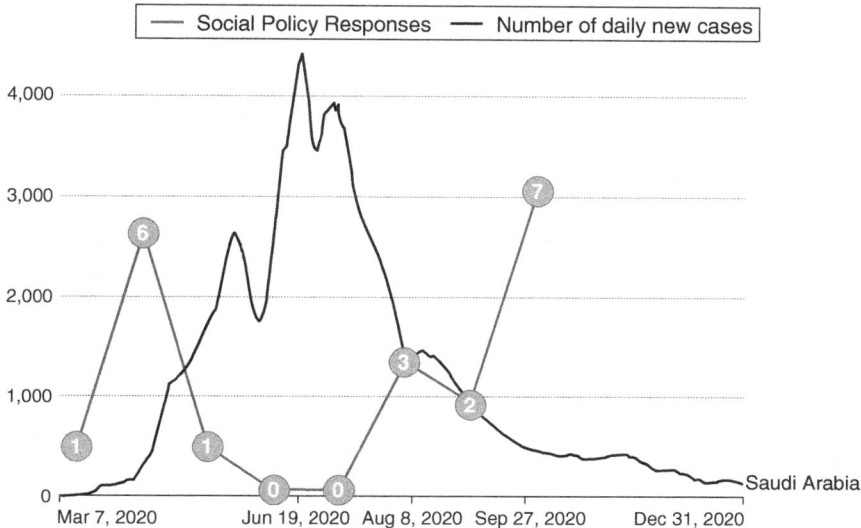

Figure 9.14 Sixth trajectory of social policy responses and number of daily new cases in Saudi Arabia, March–December 2020

The emerging need for social policy responses has been compounded by the COVID-19 pandemic, which has impacted the MENA region as much as of the rest of the world. The majority of governments implemented a shock-responsive scale-up of social policy responses, to deliver benefits in cash or in-kind, provided for children basic education, wage subsidies, short-time work schemes, and other employment or income retention measures, allowances, and/or grants aimed to support vulnerable groups against the consequences of COVID-19, benefits provided in order to ensure food security and adequate nutrition within households, benefits which are provided to families to help meet costs and needs related to child-rearing and the support of other dependents, or benefits paid to retired persons, survivors or persons with disabilities.

Conclusions

All 12 countries of our sample followed the WHO's guidance regarding the adoption of evidence-based and tested measures in the public health field. In a pandemic, the gold standard of early intervention, particularly when no effective medication or vaccine is available, is a mix of policies that aim to "flatten the curve" of daily new infections within a given territory and limit cross-boundary transmission. In this regard, it is crucial to launch a whole set of evidence-based measures early and quickly. As above-mentioned results and findings show, the countries in our sample all embarked on some sort of comprehensive policy mix based on WHO's guidance but the timing (early onset, agility), stringency, and intensity, as well as the follow-through (sustainability) of these measures varied widely across the sample and over time for almost each of the countries. Policy transfer and diffusion was an important approach used by countries, particularly within a region such as MENA, where many socio-cultural and socio-political properties are comparable.

As a result of the above-mentioned economic policy responses, particularly fiscal and monetary supports, and the successful rollout of Covid-19 vaccines in some countries in the region, economic activities have increased, which, in turn, increased oil demand and prices and put many economies on a path to recovery. However, the speed of recovery across the region will likely diverge depending on the pace of vaccination rollouts and further developments in the oil market. Oil exporting countries will likely have a faster recovery due to higher rates of inoculation and the increase in oil demand globally that brought oil prices up to pre-Covid levels and also had spillover effects on non-oil sectors. On the other hand, non-oil exporting countries that rely more on travel and tourism will likely have a slower recovery.

A major need in the context of the pandemic relates to the protection of migrant workers working in precarious forms of employment, refugees, and workers in the informal sectors across the region. Therefore, comprehensive social policy strategies that include informal workers, refugees, and migrant workers in national social policy responses, in line with international human rights and international labor standards, will play an important role in mitigating the effects of COVID-19 and support a swifter recovery. Expanding the social protection system to provide more support to vulnerable groups could be an important pillar of a "building back fairer strategy." Future research could help provide precious detailed and comparable information on financing sources and modalities, such as studies to (i) clarify the level of financing and standardize templates and definitions of financing sources; (ii) enhance our understanding of the composition of social policy financed during both the pandemic and non-crisis times; and (iii) document how successful countries have pursued a sustainable mix of financing modalities. Combined, these initiatives would help in enhancing accountability and evidence-based policymaking.

Note

1 The research for this project was supported by the Qatar National Research Fund, Rapid Response Call, Project ID RRC-7-004. We would like to thank Salman Khan, Ayah Deif, Tekla Gagoshidze, Athar Kamal, and Noureddine Radouai for their technical and research support.

References

Armingeon, K., & Beyeler, M. (2004). *The OECD and European Welfare States.* Cheltenham, Edward Elgar.

Arndt, C., & Oman, C. (2008). *The Politics of Governance Ratings.* Working Paper MGSoG/2008/WP003. Maastricht: Maastricht University, Maastricht Graduate School of Governance.

Bouckaert, G., & Van Dooren, W. (2016). Performance measurement and management in public sector organizations. In T. Bovaird & E. Loeffler (Eds.), *Public Management and Governance* (3rd ed., pp. 148–161). London: Routledge.

Bradley, C. G. (2015). International organizations and the production of indicators: The case of Freedom House. In S. E. Merry, K. E. Davis, & B. Kingsbury (Eds.), *The Quiet Power of Indicators: Measuring Governance, Corruption, and Rule of Law* (pp. 27–74). Cambridge: Cambridge University Press.

Brinks, D., & Coppedge, M. (2006). Diffusion is no illusion: Neighbor emulation in the third wave of democracy. *Comparative Political Studies*, 39(4), 463–489.

Buduru, B., & Pal, L. A. (2010). The globalized state: Measuring and monitoring governance. *European Journal of Cultural Studies*, 13(4), 511–530.

Davis, K. E., Fisher, A., Kingsbury, B., & Merry, S. E. (Eds.). (2012). *Governance by Indicators: Global Power through Classification and Rankings.* Oxford: Oxford University Press and the Institute for International Law and Justice, New York University School of Law.

Esping-Andersen, G. (1990). *The Three Worlds of Welfare Capitalism.* Cambridge: Polity Press.

Global Happiness Council. (2018). *Global Happiness Policy Report 2018.* Dubai: World Governance Summit. Available at: https://s3.amazonaws.com/ghc-2018/GlobalHappinessPolicyReport2018.pdf

Hale T., Webster S., Petherick A., Phillips T., & Kira, B. (2020). *Oxford COVID-19 government response tracker (OxCGRT)*. Blavatnik School of Government, Oxford, UK. https://www.bsg.ox.ac.uk/research/research-projects/covid-19-government-response-tracker

Helliwell, J., Layard, R., & Sachs, J. (2019). *World Happiness Report 2019*. New York: Sustainable Development Solutions Network. Available at: https://world-happiness.report/ed/2019/

Karabell, Z. (2014). *The Leading Indicators: A Short History of the Numbers that Rule Our World*. New York: Simon and Schuster.

Kaufmann, D., Kraay, A., & Mastruzzi, M. (2010). *The World Wide Governance Indicators: Methodology and Analytical Issues*. Washington, DC: The World Bank. Available at: http://papers.ssrn.com/sol3/papers.cfm?abstract_id=1682130

Leeson, P. T., & Dean, A. M. (2009). The democratic domino theory: An empirical investigation. *American Journal of Political Science*, *53*(3), 533–551. https://doi.org/10.1111/j.1540-5907.2009.00385.x

Maggetti, M., & Gilardi, F. (2016). Porblems (and solutions) in the measurement of policy diffusion mechanisms. *Journal of Public Policy*, *36*(1), 87–107. doi:10.1017/S0143814X1400035X

Merry, S. E., Davis, K. E., & Kingsbury, B. (Eds.). (2015). *The Quiet Power of Indicators: Measuring Governance, Corruption, and Rule of Law*. Cambridge: Cambridge University Press.

Mungiu-Pippidi, A. (2015). *The Quest for Good Governance: How Societies Develop Control of Corruption*. Cambridge: Cambridge University Press.

Mungiu-Pippidi, A., & Dadašov, R. (2016). Measuring control of corruption by a new index of public integrity. *European Journal on Criminal Policy Research*, *22*(3), 415–438. doi:10.1007/s10610-016-9324-z

Mungiu-Pippidi, A., & Johnston, M. (Eds.). (2017). *Transitions to Good Governance: Creating Virtuous Circles of Anti-Corruption*. Cheltenham : Edward Elgar.

New Climate Institute. (n.d.). *Climate Action Tracker*. https://climateactiontracker.org/.

Pal, L. A., & Ireland, D. (2009). The public sector reform movement: Mapping the global policy network. *International Journal of Public Administration*, *32*(8), 621–657.

Pollitt, C. (2011). Performance blight and the tyranny of light?: Accountability in advanced performance measurement regimes. In M. J. Dubnick & H. G. Frederickson (Eds.) *Accountable Governance: Problems and Promises* (pp. 81–97). Armonk, NY: M. E. Sharpe.

Raudla, R., Douglas, J. W., Randma-Liiv, T., & Savi, R. (2015). The impact of fiscal crisis on decision-making processes in European governments: Dynamics of a centralization cascade. *Public Administration Review*, *75*(6), 842–852. doi:10.1111/puar.12381

Rechkemmer, A., Ozturk, O., Brik, A. B. & Pal, L. A. (2020). COVID-19 policy tracker: MENA government responses to the crisis. www.menatracker.org

Rotberg, R. I., & Bhushan, A. (2015). The indexes of governance. In R. I. Rotberg (Ed.)*On Governance: What It Is, What It Measures and Its Policy Uses* (pp. 55–89). Waterloo: Centre for International Governance Innovation.

Rottenburg, R., Merry, S. E., Park, S.-J., & Mugler, J. (Eds.). (2015). *The World of Indicators: The Making of Governmental Knowledge Through Quanitification*. Cambridge: Cambridge University Press.

Schelkle, W. (2012). *Collapsing Worlds and Varieties of Welfare Capitalism: In Search of a New Political Economy of Welfare*. LSE Europe in Question Discussion Paper Series No. 54/2012. London: London School of Economics.

Sebhatu, A., Wennberg, K., Arora-Jonsson, S., & Lindberg, S. I. (2020). Explaining the homogeneous diffusion of COVID-19 nonpharmaceutical interventions across heterogeneous countries. *Proceedings of the National Academy of Sciences*, *117*(35), 21201–21208. https://doi.org/10.1073/pnas.2010625117

Stiglitz, J. E., Fitoussi, J.-P., & Durand, M. (2018). *Beyond GDP: Measuring What Counts for Economic and Social Performance*. Paris: OECD.

World Health Organization. (2020). Clinical management of COVID-19: Interim guidance, 27 May 2020. World Health Organization. https://apps.who.int/iris/handle/10665/332196. License: CC BY-NC-SA 3.0 IGO

10 Conclusion

The Long Shadow of Pandemic in the MENA Region: Legacy and Hope

Anis Ben Brik

Introduction

The risks and challenges posed by Covid-19 were neither unprecedented nor unexpected. They were predictable and even foreseen. Pandemics have happened many times in human history, but they are not random occurrences. For example, Thucydides provides a general account of the early stages of the plague that struck Athens in 430-426 BC in his book *History of the Peloponnesian War* (Thucydides, 1919). The declining capacity of institutions to limit misconduct and opportunistic behaviors was highlighted by Thucydides. He then goes on to discuss the consequences of the current political situation for the plague. He starts his discussion of lawlessness with the laws that were most directly violated as a result of the disaster's unique characteristics; it may also matter that these were sacred laws (Littman, 2009).

In his collection of novels *The Decameron*, the Italian writer and poet Giovanni Boccaccio (1313–1375) provided an extraordinary description of the social effects of the plague's epidemic, also known as the "Black Death," which spread throughout Italy and Mediterranean Europe during the fourteenth century (Boccaccio, 1986). Social, political, and religious institutions and hierarchies that served to organize and direct people's lives had all crumbled in Boccaccio's hometown of Florence, as they had in cities across Europe. Institutions have crumbled. Political organizations have disintegrated. Society had imploded (Perciaccante et al., 2021).

Alessandro Manzoni (1785–1873), an Italian poet and novelist, in his historical novel "*The Betrothed*" (first published in 1827) describes the same social effects of an epidemic that Boccaccio describes in his work (Bentley, 1834). Manzoni's account of the plague epidemic that ravaged Milan in 1630 is extraordinary for the level of detail it contains. After an initial lack of concern and dismissal of any warnings about plague's potential spread ("They heard with a smile of incredulity and contempt any who hazard a word on danger, or who even mentioned plague."), the novelist shows how people's fear and stigmatization of those infected with the disease evolved into a more widespread sense of "wickedness" (Perciaccante et al., 2021).

DOI: 10.4324/9781003266259-10

Albert Camus (1913–1960) provided a more recent literary account of an outbreak in his 1947 book *The Plague* (Camus, 1948). Despite being set in the 1940s, the novel is based on the cholera epidemic that struck Oran, Algeria, in 1849 following French colonization. As Camus points out in his essay, even though epidemics occur regularly, the population is always caught off guard by them. Even though everyone knows that pestilences are a fact of life, we find it hard to believe that they suddenly appear out of nowhere (Perciaccante et al., 2021). SARS, Ebola, the H1N1 flu virus, MERS, and Covid-19 have all been major epidemics in the last two decades.

The pandemic proved to be the ultimate test of the fine line between knowledge and ignorance, truth and deception, as well as the limits of greed and compassion. It was. New questions arose as countries began to regain control of the crisis: how can we reestablish a collective sense of well-being? How should we live now? Should we have compassion for anyone or anything in particular? Moreover, how should society be structured after the pandemic has passed? What would it take to get things moving again in society? As the world becomes more global, pandemics, such as COVID-19, have a long and rich history in literature.

The book's chapters examine MENA countries' responses to the pandemic and the challenges confronting the state, governance, systems, and society. While the chapters speak for themselves, we want to take a step back and survey the field in a broader context. What are the pandemic's implications for the future of the MENA region's state and society?

The Perfect Storm

This chapter went to press in early 2022, when it was estimated by the Johns Hopkins COVID-19 Dashboard that the pandemic had infected over 400 million people worldwide, with nearly 6 million deaths.[1] The MENA region had accumulated more than 13 million confirmed cases with nearly a quarter-million deaths (World Bank, 2021) causing the biggest downturn that MENA countries have ever seen. Governments have prepared for a tropical storm, but it increasingly looks like the black death plague.

The pandemic exposed serious fault lines and vulnerabilities in MENA societies, institutions, and economies. Additionally, the crisis has exacerbated several decades-old problems. These include insecurity and conflict; inequalities; unemployment; poverty; insufficient social safety nets; human rights; insufficiently responsive institutions and governance systems; and an economic model that has yet to meet universal aspirations. The urgency of the situation in MENA is heightened further by the presence of long-standing conflicts and regional divisions, which have harmed state capacity and health provision in some cases and diminished prospects for effective regional cooperation. It is particularly acute in countries already afflicted by conflict or economic crisis. Libya and Iraq, for example, are still suffering from the effects of war and weakened infrastructure – in April and June

2021, two major fires swept through critical hospital facilities in Iraq, killing at least 200 people (Alsabri et al., 2021).

Yemen has been dubbed the world's worst humanitarian disaster, with 80% of the population in need of assistance, though the pandemic ranks lower on the threat scale when compared to widespread hunger and other diseases (Fawcett, 2021). In Syria, the ongoing war has resulted in the closure of up to 40% of hospitals and primary care facilities; many healthcare workers are refugees or internally displaced. Lebanon, which is currently undergoing an economic and political crisis, suffered a massive explosion in August 2020 in the capital's port area, reducing hospital capacity by more than 30%; Iran is subject to US economic sanctions, which restrict its ability to access vital equipment and medicines (Fawcett, 2021).

Along with the COVID-19 crisis, the region was hit by a second shock when oil prices plummeted to their lowest level in 17 years. State revenues in the region are reliant on oil, and if prices remained near $20 a barrel, Gulf countries faced a daily loss of $554 million (Strategy&, 2021). Additionally, wars and conflict pose a significant impediment to responding to COVID-19, putting millions of people in far more precarious situations than they would have been otherwise, from a health, humanitarian, human rights, and socioeconomic standpoint (PwC, 2021).

The MENA region was already one of the most unequal regions in the world in terms of wealth distribution; the pandemic exacerbated the problem. The poor are particularly vulnerable to the disease's ravages, and poor countries are less equipped to contain it (OECD, 2020a). The pandemic brought the negative consequences of violence and conflict into sharper focus. Widespread inequality, mass unemployment, underdeveloped social safety nets, human rights violations, and poor governance have exacerbated the epidemiological challenges in several of the region's war-torn societies (UN, 2020a,b).

The region's most vulnerable and impoverished countries now face severe social dislocation, recession, and increased political instability (Roger, 2020). Furthermore, much of the MENA region's labor markets are precarious and informal, at least for those who do not work directly for the state or large firms. Typically, the informal sector pays lower wages, and workers lack the social protections and insurance benefits available to those employed in the formal sector. Thus, the spread of COVID-19 and lockdowns have taken a heavy toll on the region's most vulnerable informal workers. Many have been laid off and have few alternative sources of income. This is not merely a humanitarian crisis; it also poses a serious threat to social and political stability.

Health Preparedness

COVID-19 is afflicting the MENA region at a time where health care in many countries is fragmented and primary care is underserved. The pandemic has highlighted the deep inequalities and uneven capacity of health systems. One-third of Arab countries have fewer than ten healthcare providers per 10,000 people, while the richest third have at least 50 providers per 10,000 population and, in some cases, over 70.9. The regional doctor-to-population ratio stands at 2.9 per 1,000 people, below the world ratio of 3.42 per 1,000 people (UN, 2020a,b). COVID-19 is wreaking havoc in the MENA region at a time when health care is fragmented and primary care is underserved in many countries. The pandemic has brought to light the system's profound inequalities and disparities. One-third of MENA countries have fewer than ten healthcare providers per 10,000 people, while the richest third have at least 50 and, in some cases, more than 70.9 providers per 10,000 people. The regional doctor-to-population ratio is 2.9 doctors for every 1,000 people, which is lower than the global ratio of 3.42 doctors for every 1,000 people (UN, 2020a,b).

Many countries in the MENA region are ill-prepared to deal with a pandemic. Healthcare systems are frail, infrastructure is inadequate, and there are far too few providers of health care. In general, hospitalization and mortality rates have been lower in the region than in other regions, owing in part to the region's very young population. With nearly 60% of the population under the age of 25, MENA is one of the world's most youthful regions (OECD, 2020). However, it is also one of the most unequal, with significant socioeconomic consequences in terms of lost GDP, food insecurity, interruptions to education, and unemployment, as well as the impact on vulnerable communities such as migrant workers and refugees. Furthermore, healthcare systems remain deficient, even in the wealthiest states; the region as a whole lags behind comparable peers (OECD, 2020a). Health expenditures range from 0.6% of GDP in Yemen to 4.6% in Palestine (Talbot, 2020). Due to significant differences in data collection methods and state capacity, it is difficult to compare morbidity and case statistics across the region. Certain countries do not publish morbidity data, and COVID-19 testing is not administered uniformly throughout the region (Roger, 2020). These shortcomings have resulted in a serious regional transparency crisis with negative public health, social, and economic consequences. By and large, wealthier countries are far better equipped to generate trustworthy public health data, administer virus testing, and enforce effective public health regulations (Roger, 2020). The most destabilized countries are in a much worse position. Yemen, a war-torn and impoverished country, has simply ceased publishing testing data, and there are signs that COVID-19 rates in that country are skyrocketing. Syria, the densely populated Gaza Strip, and Libya are all ill-equipped to deal with this public health crisis (Roger, 2020).

Youth

The MENA region has a very young population, and those under the age of 30 are particularly resilient to COVID-19's most severe physical effects.

However, as a result of this pandemic, young people face additional socio-economic burdens. Over the last quarter-century, the region's youth unemployment rate has remained consistently above 25%, compared to a global average of 13%. (Roger, 2020). The MENA region had the highest rate of youth unemployment in the world in 2019, although the figures varied significantly. The Arab Spring was partially a response to young people's profound dissatisfaction with the region's political and economic systems. Activists charged that ruling elite were systematic in their denial of economic opportunity and adequate political expression to young people. The situation has deteriorated significantly (Roger, 2020).

Refugees

MENA is home to millions of internally displaced people and refugees, with camps in Jordan, Iraq, Lebanon, and Syria adding to the strain on already-fragile infrastructure. Although data on refugee camps remain scarce, scholars have highlighted the additional challenges posed by the pandemic in protecting the rights of vulnerable refugee populations in host countries that restrict movement and access (Barnes and Makinda, 2021). The region's refugee communities are particularly vulnerable on this front due to substandard housing, overcrowding, and insufficient health care. Even prior to the pandemic, meeting the needs of refugees in Lebanon and Jordan became more difficult due to medical service and supply shortages. By autumn 2020, the vulnerability of the region's estimated 15 million refugees and internally displaced persons became clear as the COVID-19 epidemic swept through several of these communities (Fawcett, 2021). Infection rates in Syrian, Iraqi, Lebanese, and Palestinian refugee camps increased significantly in September.

Women

Women are especially vulnerable to an economic downturn in the informal sector, where they account for 61.8% of workers (UN, 2020a,b). The burden is compounded by the fact that women are typically responsible for children who are unable to attend school due to widespread lockdowns. In much of the region, women face systematic job discrimination and are over-represented among the unemployed. Women in the region have the lowest formal labor force participation rate (20%) in the world, owing in part to discriminatory social norms. They entered the current crisis already in precarious circumstances, and the crisis has only exacerbated their predicament (OECD, 2020b).

Policy Responses

Against the above backdrop, MENA countries implemented early policy responses that successfully 'flattened the curve.' By early March 2020, as the threat of infection became clear, the region's governments began implementing significant containment measures, including travel restrictions and school, factory, and store closures. Border closures on a limited scale ensued, jeopardizing trade and supply chains. Additionally, places of worship have been closed, and several countries have invoked emergency legislation to impose quarantine measures on the general public. Certain governments have declared states of emergency, public health emergencies, and national disasters. Declaring a state of emergency confers expanded authority on governments, frequently including the authority to restrict movement, prohibit public gatherings, and impose curfews. In some instances, governments have invoked a state of emergency to monitor communications, censor media content, and detain individuals deemed to be a threat to "national security." Violations of emergency-related orders frequently face stiff monetary fines or imprisonment, further restricting an already restrictive environment for human rights and civic space in MENA. In response to COVID outbreaks, several countries have implemented partial or general curfews (Table 10.1).

While the Covid-19 pandemic is still unfolding, striking differences in MENA countries' responses and outcomes are already evident. States' approaches to disease management range from repression to mitigation and accommodation. Additionally, they differ in the methods used to accomplish these goals, ranging from direct enforcement via regulatory directives and criminal sanctions to more indirect encouragement and persuasion.

Policy Responses in the Gulf Region

At the outset of the COVID-19 crisis, promising initiatives included the establishment of a Gulf crisis room to coordinate responses and a network to

Table 10.1 MENA policy responses to the pandemic

Measures	Countries
State of Emergency	Palestine, Mauritania, Tunisia, Morocco, Egypt
Public Health Emergencies	Sudan, Lebanon
Activation of a National Defense Law	Jordan
Curfew and Lockdowns	Algeria, Egypt, Iran, Iraq, Jordan, Kuwait, Lebanon, Morocco, Oman, Qatar, Saudi Arabia, Tunisia, UAE
Banning the printing and sale of newspapers	Jordan, Algeria, UAE, Oman, Morocco, Saudi Arabia, Yemen
Legal measures to counter "fake news"	Morocco, Jordan, Egypt, Oman, the UAE
Surveillance technology	Oman, UAE, Bahrain, Saudi Arabia, Jordan, Kuwait, Qatar, Tunisia, Morocco

Source: Honstein (2021).

safeguard food supplies – a critical area given the region's reliance on external food supply chains (Rossi and Kabbani, 2020). From a health standpoint, one critical factor is the gulf countries' prior exposure to MERS, a virus transmitted to humans via infected camels that were first reported in 2012, with Saudi Arabia being the most affected state. Assembly bans have also impacted religious gatherings: Saudi Arabia's authorities have restricted the annual pilgrimage to Mecca to an estimated 1,000 residents, despite the event's tradition of attracting approximately 2 million Muslims from around the world (Karadsheh and Qiblawi, 2020).

The pandemic has exposed the vulnerability of certain segments of the Gulf population, particularly migrant workers, who frequently live in more crowded and unsanitary conditions with unequal access to health care (Karasapan, 2020). The absence of a regional mechanism to manage migration and labor conditions for such informal workers (many of whom are women) had been a source of concern long before COVID struck, but the pandemic has brought their plight into sharper focus, with evidence also indicating that mortality rates among migrant workers have been significantly higher than those among local populations (Fawcett, 2021).

Policy Responses in the Levant Region

Jordan's response to the pandemic has been robust, despite criticism of its aggressive policing of lockdowns and borders; Syria remains a war-torn country with scant data on the pandemic's impact. However, Medecins Sans Frontieres (MSF) reported on the severity of a new wave that hit Northern Syria in October 2021 (MSF, 2021). Curfews remained in place in Egypt and Jordan until July 2020, but on a reduced and fluctuating basis based on virus-related indicators, such as the number of new cases per day. Other countries have enacted legislation prohibiting public gatherings. In Iraq, for example, the Supreme Committee for National Health and Safety has prohibited all types of gatherings and imposed stiff penalties on violators (Fawcett, 2021).

Policy Responses in North African Countries

Algeria, Morocco, and Tunisia have all taken extensive measures to contain the virus, which has had a detrimental effect on their economies and, in the case of Tunisia, contributed to sustained political unrest, but despite the region's gravity, its members have been unable to put aside political differences to support a common approach. In July/August 2021, the region experienced a high caseload and, despite a subsequent decline, Libya continued to experience high rates of infection and uneven vaccination rates. Algeria and Libya had fully vaccinated only 13% and 15% of their respective populations, compared to significantly higher rates in Morocco (65%) and Tunisia (40%), respectively (Reuters, 2020).

Policy Responses in Iran

Iran's situation is particularly complicated due to the pandemic's rapid on-set and severity, its relative regional and global isolation in the face of ongoing conflicts with Arab states, Israel, and the West, and the punitive effects of US sanctions. While Iran's health sector is relatively developed, as is its research and technology base, the country's economy is particularly vulnerable as a result of the pandemic's scope, the effects of falling oil prices, and international sanctions restricting the country's access to currency and vital supplies. While Iran has implemented a variety of lockdown and preventive measures, some of which have been delayed due to the March Nowruz (New Year) celebrations, the country remains the worst-affected MENA country. It has previously relied on vaccine supplies from China, Russia, and India, as well as the COVAX program, but initial vaccination rates have been low – approximately 5% in July 2021 (ReliefWeb, 2020).

Digital Technologies' Responses

Many countries in the MENA region have relied on surveillance technology to assist in tracking and preventing the virus's spread. The Gulf countries made extensive use of cutting-edge technology, with Qatar launching a nationwide coronavirus tracking app called Ehteraz and the UAE launching a mass drive-through testing program. Nabta, Kuwait's new women's health-care app, also provides users with up-to-date information on COVID-related health issues (Al-Hosani et al., 2021).

Oman and Tunisia have both used drones and robots to monitor the movement of quarantine individuals and impose restrictions on social gatherings. The UAE, Bahrain, Saudi Arabia, Jordan, Kuwait, Qatar, Tunisia, and Morocco have all adopted new contact-tracing apps. Jordan, for example, mandated the use of a COVID-19 tracing app for all government employees and anyone who visits a government agency. It is still unknown whether the use of such technology is effective in containing the virus's spread, and concerns are growing about the technology's negative impact on the right to privacy and the protection of personal data (Honstein, 2021).

Theories and Practices

The pandemic has been a stress test for our theories. It has both elevated new research questions and compelled us to reconsider some established theoretical approaches. In this section, we return to theory and consider some of the institutional learning lessons that have been observed thus far around Covid-19, as well as the crisis's implications for theories and practices.

Analyzing the COVID-19 pandemic's effect through a philosophical lens can provide insight and discovery into new perspectives on this watershed year. Michel Foucault's work, in particular, can provide theories and explanations for the effect of mass vaccination and government intervention on a population.

Biopolitics

Examining the COVID-19 pandemic through a Foucauldian lens necessitates the application of Foucault's theories and concepts. Governments have enforced mask mandates and distancing regulations to prolong human life and ensure the population's safety by preventing the state body from becoming ill and dying in large numbers. Vaccination is a subset of biopolitics in which governments actively exert control over their populations by ensuring their survival. Additionally, vaccines represent an intense form of institutional power, as governments gain the ability to determine who lives and who dies by making decisions about which groups within society must be vaccinated first. Foucault's concept of biopolitics enables us to comprehend how the government's inequitable distribution of vaccines is literally resulting in the deaths of marginalized people. We are witnessing biopolitics at its most heinous, in which a state possesses the ability to provide for its unified body but fails to do so due to internal and systemic problems (Hubbard, 2021).

Governmentality

COVID-19 contact tracing is also better understood in light of Foucault's 'Governmentality' theory. Governmentality, as defined by Foucault, is the union of two forces – government and rationality – that enables governments to direct and shape the behavior of their citizens. The scientific and medical community's promotion of awareness and protection within society influenced a shift in human behavior, as individuals were forced to become more aware of their own well-being. Yet, two years into the pandemic, MENA populations have accepted mask mandates; while they may not personally enjoy or support them, they recognize that the mandates have become ingrained in daily life. Tracking the rise of the mask mandate and individuals' views on them over time allows us to gain a better understanding of governmentality as a whole and how institutions can influence society's behavior (Hubbard, 2021).

Disciplinary Power

Foucault's creation of the concept of 'disciplinary power' is another aspect of his philosophy that can explain phenomena resulting from the COVID-19 pandemic. Throughout the COVID-19 pandemic, we have witnessed governments use the concept of disciplinary power to alter their citizens' behavior and help stop the spread of the pandemic. The normalization of masks and social distancing are examples of this power at work. Throughout the pandemic, we have also witnessed the power institutions hold in determining the outcome of our lives and our manner of behavior (Hubbard, 2021).

Another aspect of Foucault's philosophy that can be used to explain the COVID-19 pandemic is the concept of 'disciplinary power.' Throughout the COVID-19 pandemic, governments have used the concept of disciplinary power to influence their citizens' behavior and aid in the pandemic's containment. The normalization of masks and social distancing are both manifestations of this power. We have also witnessed the power institutions wield in determining the outcome of our lives and our behavior throughout the pandemic (Hubbard, 2021).

The Roles of the State

The history of epidemic control teaches us that debates over the appropriate balance of state enforcement and community self-organization are not novel. The extent to which the Derbyshire village of Eyam, whose population self-isolated when the plague spread from London in 1665, demonstrates that towns and villages were not uncommon at the time, and were sometimes imposed entirely through community action, has been questioned (Deakin and Meng, 2020).

We are all now statists. Since the coronavirus pandemic struck and destabilized the global economy, we have looked to governments to mobilize medical resources, implement containment measures, and spend previously unimaginable sums to assist workers and businesses. These emergency policies may result in the establishment of new institutions and methods of problem-solving that will benefit us long after the pandemic has passed. There is also a dark side. Governments have expanded their capabilities for tracing, tracking, and controlling. Several of them have already abused these authorities, and it is entirely possible that they will never relinquish them (Crabtree et al., 2020).

Crabtree et al. (2020) argue that the pandemic has focused attention on a number of issues, including corruption, transparency, accountability, information, trust, digitalization, and governance, and unsurprisingly, the debate has produced several conundrums:

- Accountability and transparency: As states respond to demands, communication must be open and transparent in order to foster trust. Yet, when transparency is present but not accompanied by accountability, people become more cynical and frustrated.
- Infodemic. States have a role to play in a crisis in terms of harnessing technology for the benefit of citizens and acting as honest broker of what information is truly relevant.
- Public confidence. A balance between top-down support and investments in lower-level expertise is required. Local institutions can compensate for a lack of trust in or frustration with national institutions.

- Digital capital. Numerous questions have been raised about the location and pace of digital capital. It is critical to prioritize digital infrastructure for critical services. Nonetheless, significant disparities in digital access exist across the MENA region.
- Corruption and governance: States must also address legalized corruption and misgovernance. Policy analysts and activists could use this lens to diagnose and counter inaction or self-serving public health responses and economic stimuli in a pandemic context.

The state's capacity, as the 'focal' or 'sovereign' agent, to retrieve, store, and disseminate information derived from social and customary practices becomes a critical determinant of effective pandemic responses. The state's role in this process is to stabilize norms and alter social practices by altering perceptions of what constitutes normatively appropriate behavior and by rebalancing the costs and benefits associated with compliance with the legal system's publicly enunciated standards (Deakin and Meng, 2020).

The question is whether this represents an "authoritarian temptation" or an "authoritarian moment," or something more benign, such as a more robust state reshaping the economy and society for the benefit of its citizens. We may see a trend toward "soft securitization," in which continuous but low-level and deferential monitoring, checking, confirming, reconfirming, measuring, assessing, and reporting occur (Pal and Ben Brik, 2021). As previously stated, the pandemic's impact on states and institutions will be ambiguous. On the one hand, despite the immediate role of nation-states in containing the pandemic on the ground, the crisis should serve as a reminder of the critical nature of institutions and governance. There are two potential sleeper issues: one that awoke unexpectedly in the summer of 2022 and another that is likely to emerge in 2023. The latter refers to fiscal constraints and deficits (Pal and Ben Brik, 2021).

The Future

Despite the pandemic's protracted and devastating nature, the increase in vaccination rates and the development of effective treatments have allowed us to look forward with some optimism. However, as we begin to see the light at the end of the tunnel, it is critical to recognize the various ways in which MENA governments can rebuild more effectively.

With contact tracing becoming routine and vaccination becoming more widespread, significant barriers to privacy protection have fallen and will be difficult to rebuild. Whether the pandemic is eradicated or persists, it exposed a slew of festering issues, most painfully in unstable countries, but also in other MENA countries where people suffered corrupt or inept governments (Pal and Ben Brik, 2021). Public health services, income inequality, social media pathologies, gender, the competence of government institutions, freedom and human rights, authoritarianism, trust in governments, and the digital divide became daily, tumultuous, and occasionally perplexing topics of discussion. The pandemic appeared to expose a fatal flaw in long-accepted economic, political, and institutional structures.

The Future of the State

The coronavirus pandemic is highlighting the inadequacy of governments worldwide. It is expected to usher in a new era of larger, more intrusive government in nearly every advanced economy – but most notably in the majority of MENA countries. Gulf countries have moved quickly to increase spending, protecting citizens and businesses through wage support programs and cash payouts. This is especially true in Qatar, Saudi Arabia, Kuwait, Bahrain, Oman, and the UAE, which have long taken pride in their relatively large governments.

MENA countries will undoubtedly require larger governments as they scramble to develop expansive new tools for disease control, workplace management, and social surveillance in the hope of containing future outbreaks. Again, given their resources, Gulf countries are likely to take the lead in this area. In short, the era of a large government is returning, but in ways that are quite different from the 1960s and 1970s era of large states (Walt and Belfer, 2020).

States that are responsive, data-driven, energetic, collaborative, and innovative will outperform autocracies in defending their societies against the coronavirus and its economic costs – leaving these governments strengthened and enjoying increased public trust in the future (Wrage, 2020).

Future of Governance

Infectious disease outbreaks have had a profound effect on public governance throughout history. In the fourteenth century, the bubonic plague prompted a rethinking of squalid urban spaces. In the nineteenth century, cholera outbreaks sparked massive urban redevelopment projects and a dramatic expansion of sewage systems (Crabtree et al., 2020). The current coronavirus pandemic will also result in significant changes in governance – from the use of invasive surveillance technologies to track infections and enforce quarantines to increased healthcare spending to combat this and future diseases (Muggah, 2020).

The COVID-19 pandemic in MENA has exposed the region's contrasting strengths and weaknesses in governance. Examining how countries have responded to pandemics can help governments improve their ability to respond in the future. Numerous MENA countries, including those endowed with natural resources, exhibit lax – and frequently deteriorating – governance standards, including leadership failures; a loss of "voice" and accountability; and, consequently, high levels of corruption and capture by political and economic elites. Yet, governance matters more than ever right now: countries with higher governance standards are responding and coping better with the pandemic than countries with low governance standards (Kaufmann, 2020).

MENA governments are likely to face several significant challenges regardless of their preparations. Coordination and communication across levels of government will need to be effective if the response is to be successful. This holds both for information sharing about disease spread from local communities to the central government and vice versa. Another complicating factor will be the pandemic's international spread. As previously stated, states and local communities will be called upon to act as first responders in the event of a pandemic. They, in turn, will need to rely more heavily on individual social responsibility and assistance to respond more effectively.

The omicron wave once again demonstrates the MENA countries' vulnerability to the crisis. This vulnerability underscores the critical nature of governments treating serious outbreaks as security threats and prioritizing the protection of their populations. Omicron increased booster to use in high-income countries, created confusion about the efficacy of existing vaccines, and complicated vaccination campaigns in MENA. Omicron and the emergence of additional variants may also make it more difficult for countries to reach an agreement on pandemic governance reforms, such as concluding a pandemic treaty or instrument, increasing vaccine production capacity, or resolving patent disputes (Coggi and Regazzoni, 2022). Finally, public fear management will be a critical component of the government's response (Cook and Cohen, 2008).

Future of Social Welfare

The pandemic has disproportionately impacted the poor and vulnerable in MENA, in large part due to historically limited coverage of social safety nets and a deteriorating situation even prior to COVID-19. The crises were largely precipitated by oil price declines, institutional fragility, and conflict in a number of countries, most notably Yemen, Syria, Libya, and Iraq. Internally displaced persons and refugees have been further exposed to extreme vulnerability as a result of illness and the loss of informal sector employment opportunities. Social safety nets have been shown to be extremely effective at mitigating the crisis's impact and fostering resilience, even among the poorest households. MENA countries had previously announced a range of social protection measures to address the effects of COVID-19, including social assistance, social insurance, and labor market programs. Numerous measures are modeled after and built upon existing social protection policies, strategies, and programs. Increased coverage is accomplished through either vertical expansion, in which existing beneficiaries receive additional benefits, or horizontal expansion, in which additional beneficiaries are targeted. This magnitude demonstrates the responsiveness and scalability of MENA's social protection systems. And the emergency response pushed the social protection system to its limits by mandating the use of technology for payments, establishing and expanding the use of social registries, expanding coverage and benefits horizontally and vertically, and implementing a variety of other interventions. While the ongoing vaccination campaign will be critical in spearheading the region's recovery, social protection will be equally critical in the months and years ahead. Even as the recovery gains traction, governments will face severe fiscal constraints, forcing them to make difficult spending and policy choices. Returning to the new normal will require policy choices that address the needs of poor and vulnerable households, communities, and small businesses (Belhaj, 2021). Thus, rethinking social welfare in MENA is even more critical going forward. It will be critical to assist countries in strengthening and accelerating policy reforms and innovations that provide adequate social protection coverage for informal sector workers, reform regressive subsidies to create fiscal space for targeted social safety nets, strengthen delivery systems, and invest in institutions capable of championing the social protection agenda and guiding policy and implementation.

Regional Cooperation

The Coronavirus pandemic struck at a point in the region's history when insecurity and regional fragmentation were at an all-time high. Political divisions within the region, as well as geopolitical divisions beyond, have all hampered cooperation. Nonetheless, global health threats, like environmental threats, know no political boundaries and necessitate effective state collaboration. While sub-regions such as the Gulf, the Levant, and North Africa all present opportunities for cross-border cooperation – opportunities that are frequently overlooked – there is also a need for a broader regional framework that includes all MENA actors. Now is the time to support a renewed multilateral effort to address multiple problems, one that includes major regional and external powers, as well as international organizations. It may provide the impetus for cooperation that the region so desperately needs, by initiating a series of confidence-building measures to advance the region's limited progress thus far.

International assistance to some of the region's most vulnerable communities will be critical in the coming years, and given the global financial crisis, a reduction in such assistance appears likely. The region faces the risk of exploding if basic humanitarian needs are not met. This would have grave implications for the international community's security. Medical assistance will be critical, and once treatments or vaccines are available to help mitigate the COVID-19 crisis's impact, they should be made widely available to the region's residents. Numerous countries, including Qatar, the UAE, Kuwait, and Saudi Arabia, have taken a proactive stance on this front by donating substantial supplies of medical equipment to numerous countries throughout the region.

Due to the COVID-19 crisis, the basic needs of migrants and refugees living throughout the MENA region cannot be overlooked, and these communities will require both local and international assistance. All recovery plans must take their needs into account. The international community's priority should continue to be providing medical assistance to internally displaced persons and refugees in conflict-torn regions. Efforts to address the unique challenges that women in the MENA region face as a result of this crisis will be critical. They are the most likely to experience the crisis's social and economic consequences and will require assistance from their governments and the international community.

Conclusion

Since 2000, the MENA region has been mired in a spiral of conflict and insecurity, with new wars and divisions complicating the landscape. Along with the Israel-Palestine conflict, new issues have clogged the regional agenda, ranging from the Yemeni crisis to the Syrian conflict, the Iran-Saudi rivalry to the ongoing impasse over Iran's nuclear program, and the perfect storm of the COVID-19 pandemic. Numerous MENA countries were forced to scramble to respond, stumbled, reversed course, and made policy on the fly. While early policy responses were frequently chaotic and uncoordinated, as the crisis progressed and more information became available, and as the curve eventually flattened out by mid-summer 2021, a degree of stability in crisis response emerged. Additionally, critics have highlighted some of the negative consequences of the securitization of health policies, such as the widespread use of health apps, which have increased the power and scrutiny of centralized authoritarian regimes while limiting individual rights and freedoms.

Across MENA, policy responses came in four distinct and overlapping waves. The initial response was medical – caring for the sick and dying, as evidenced by grim scenes of overcrowded hospitals and intensive care units. In almost every MENA country, the second set of policy responses included a variety of non-pharmaceutical interventions ('NPIs'), such as quarantines, cordons sanitaires, and unprecedented "lockdowns" of virtually everything, from parks and schools to places of work and worship, in conjunction with unprecedented population tracing and tracking and COVID-19 testing. The third wave was "re-lockdown" in countries experiencing renewed spikes in omicron-related cases. A fourth wave that has not yet materialized is the cautious and staged "re-opening" of economies and societies.

The pandemic's greatest conundrum was the trade-off between public health and economic recovery. Lockdowns and other necessary public health measures to contain the virus triggered a severe economic downturn across the region, with the World Bank forecasting an average regional GDP growth rate of 4.2% in 2022 if the pandemic recedes and obscures individual country differences (World Bank, 2022).

Literature can teach us valuable lessons about the past, and it should also help us live a better life in the present. However, by examining historical examples of epidemics, including fictionalized accounts of historical epidemics, we can conclude that the current pandemic demonstrates that the responses to an unknown disease have been reported constant over time, demonstrating that "there is nothing new under the sun" (Ecclesiastes 1:9). This chapter makes the assumption that the pandemic shock will linger with us for years, reverberating through theory and practice. That shock is not entirely a shock associated with the novel crisis. While the pandemic altered the policy landscape significantly, it amplified trends and tendencies that existed prior to it or will exacerbate and infect existing debates and conflicts. Securitization is a clear example – governments have long tracked and monitored their citizens. The pandemic compelled the development of new tracking apps, increased policing, and the monitoring and lockdown of entire societies.

The Decameron teaches us that times of crisis necessitate new narratives. When an ancient world is destroyed, we must resist the temptation to recycle familiar stories or to seek refuge in predictable narrative formulas. As Boccaccio explicitly states, storytelling is a profoundly social process and practice. This is true in The Decameron in terms of storytelling context (everyone has the opportunity to tell multiple stories), storytelling form (sharing in both vernacular and prose), and storytelling content. Telling stories is a way of thinking collaboratively, reflecting collectively, and thereby establishing a new way of being with others (Perciaccante et al., 2021).

While many of us remain quarantined in a manner similar to that used during the Black Death, which stories will we hear in the coming days, weeks, and months? Additionally, and in keeping with Boccaccio's teachings, what new narratives will each of us create and share?

The "world" is a socially shared sense of belonging, reinforced by everyday institutions and rituals. When a pandemic strike, we lose our world and descend into unhealthy, prolonged periods of isolation, extreme forms of alienation, and seemingly endless angst. In the midst of a pandemic, we are acutely aware of our social nature (Poll, 2020).

But hope persists in pandemics.

Note

1 COVID-19 Dashboard by the Center for Systems Science and Engineering (CSSE) at Johns Hopkins University, https://coronavirus.jhu.edu/map.html. Another reputable source with a slightly different total (27,113,459 infected; 884,527 dead) is the CoronaTracker, available at https://www.coronatracker.com/

References

Al-Hosani, F., Al-Mazrouei, S., Al-Memari, S., Al-Yafei, Z., Paulo, M. S., & Koornneef, E. (2021). A review of COVID-19 mass testing in the United Arab Emirates. *Frontiers in Public Health*, *9*. https://doi.org/10.3389/fpubh.2021.661134

Alsabri, M., Alhadheri, A., Alsakkaf, L. M., & Cole, J. (2021). Conflict and COVID-19 in Yemen: Beyond the humanitarian crisis. *Globalization and Health*, *17*(1). https://doi.org/10.1186/s12992-021-00732-1

Barnes, J., & Makinda, S. M. (2021). A threat to cosmopolitan duties? How COVID-19 has been used as a tool to undermine refugee rights. *International Affairs, 97*(6), 1671–1689. https://doi.org/10.1093/ia/iiab156

Belhaj, F. (2021). *Social Protection for All in Need: Lessons from the COVID-19 Response in MENA.* World Bank Blogs. https://blogs.worldbank.org/arabvoices/social-protection-for-all-lessons-from-covid-19-response-mena

Bentley, R. R. (1834). Josephi Ripamontii, canoniscalensis, chronistae urbis Mediolani, de peste quae fuit anno 1630. *Libri V,* 369–400.

Boccaccio, G. (1986). *The Decameron.* New York: Black WJ Inc. Translated by John Payne; pp. 1–9.

Camus, A. (1948). *The Plague.* New York: Random House. Translated by Stuart Gilbert; pp. 1–287.

Coggi, P. T., & Regazzoni, C. J. (2022). *COVID-19 After Two Years: The Failure of Pandemic Governance.* Council of Councils, New York, US. https://www.cfr.org/councilofcouncils/global-memos/covid-19-after-two-years-failure-pandemic-governance

Cook, A. H., & Cohen, D. B. (2008). Pandemic disease: A past and future challenge to governance in the United States. *Review of Policy Research, 25*(5), 449–471. https://doi.org/10.1111/j.1541-1338.2008.00346.x

Crabtree, J., Kaplan, R. D., Muggah, R., Naidoo, K., O'Neil, S. K., Posen, A., Roth, K., Schneier, B., Walt, S. M., & Wrage, A. (2020). *The Future of the State.* Foreign Policy, Washington, D.C. https://foreignpolicy.com/2020/05/16/future-government-powers-coronavirus-pandemic/

Deakin, S., & Meng, G. (2020). The governance of COVID-19: Anthropogenic risk, evolutionary learning, and the future of the social state. *Industrial Law Journal, 49*(4), 539–594. https://doi.org/10.1093/indlaw/dwaa027

Fawcett, L. (2021). The Middle East and COVID-19: Time for collective action. *Globalization and Health, 17*(133). https://doi.org/10.1186/s12992-021-00786-1

Honstein, E. (2021). *Middle Eastern and North African Government Responses to COVID-19.* ICNL, Washington, D.C. https://www.icnl.org/post/news/mena-government-responses-to-covid-19

Hubbard, C. (2021). *What Foucault Can Teach Us About Covid-19: Understanding the Effects of the Pandemic through Philosophy.* The World Mind. https://www.theworldmind.org/home/2021/5/6/what-foucault-can-teach-us-about-covid-19-understanding-the-effects-of-the-pandemic-through-philosophy

Karadsheh, J., & Qiblawi, T. (2020). *'Unprecedented' Hajj Begins – with 1,000 Pilgrims, Rather Than the Usual 2 Million.* CNN. https://edition.cnn.com/travel/article/hajj-2020-coronavirus-intl/index.html

Karasapan, O. (2020). *Pandemic Highlights the Vulnerability of Migrant Workers in the Middle East.* Brookings, Washington, D.C. https://www.brookings.edu/blog/future-development/2020/09/17/pandemic-highlights-the-vulnerability-of-migrant-workers-in-the-middle-east/

Kaufmann, D. (2020). *What the Pandemic Reveals About Governance, State Capture, and Natural Resources.* Brookings, Washington, D.C. https://www.brookings.edu/blog/future-development/2020/07/10/what-the-pandemic-reveals-about-governance-state-capture-and-natural-resources/

Littman, R. J. (2009). The plague of Athens: Epidemiology and paleopathology. *Mount Sinai Journal of Medicine: A Journal of Translational and Personalized Medicine, 76*(5), 456–467. https://doi.org/10.1002/msj.20137

MSF. (2021). *Health System Overwhelmed in Northern Syria in Most Severe COVID-19 Outbreak Yet.* Médecins Sans Frontières (MSF) International, Dubai, UAE. https://www.msf.org/health-system-overwhelmed-northern-syria-most-severe-covid-19-outbreak-yet

Muggah, R. (2020). *Local Government Will Emerge Stronger After the Pandemic.* https://foreignpolicy.com/2020/05/16/future-government-powers-coronavirus-pandemic/.

OECD (2020a). *COVID-19 Crisis Response in MENA Countries.* https://read.oecd-ilibrary.org/view/?ref=129_129919-4li7bq8asv&title=COVID-19-Crisis-Response-in-MENA-Countries

OECD (2020b). *COVID-19 Response in MENA Countries.* https://www.oecd.org/coronavirus/policy-responses/covid-19-crisis-response-in-mena-countries-4b366396/

Pal, L. A., & Ben Brik A. (2021). *Conclusion. Future tense: A new grammar for the policy sciences? In The Future of the Policy Sciences.* Chicago, IL: Edward Elgar Publishing. 180–203.

Perciaccante, A., Malacrea, M., Coralli, A., & Donell, S. (2021). Literature "magistra vitae": What literature teaches about society's reactions to pandemic outbreaks. *Ethics, Medicine and Public Health, 18,* 100657. https://doi.org/10.1016/j.jemep.2021.100657

Poll R. (2020). *Why boccaccio's 'The Decameron' can help guide us through COVID-19. PopMatters.* https://www.popmatters.com/boccaccio-decameron-2645749241.html

PwC. (2021). *The GCC Post-Pandemic: Massive and Fast Transformation.* https://www.pwc.com/m1/en/assets/document/gcc-massive-fast-transformation-print.pdf

ReliefWeb (2020). *Islamic Republic of Iran Receives Second Delivery of COVID-19 Vaccines through the COVAX Facility - Iran.* https://reliefweb.int/report/iran-islamic-republic/islamic-republic-iran-receives-second-delivery-covid-19-vaccines

Reuters (2020). *Coronavirus in Asia and the Middle East: The Latest Counts, Charts and Maps.* https://graphics.reuters.com/world-coronavirus-tracker-and-maps/regions/asia-and-the-middle-east/

Roger, G. (2020). *The COVID-19 Pandemic and the Middle East and North Africa Region: Special Report.* Nato Parliamentary Assembly. https://www.nato-pa.int/download-file?filename=/sites/default/files/2021-01/095%20GSM%2020`20E%20rev%202%20fin-%20COVID%20PANDEMIC%20IN%20THE%20MENA%20REGION.pdf

Rossi, T., & Kabbani, N. (2020). *How Gulf States Can Lead the Global COVID-19 Response.* Brookings, Washington, D.C. https://www.brookings.edu/opinions/how-gulf-states-can-lead-the-global-covid-19-response/

Strategy& (2021). *Recovering from the Dual Shock of COVID-19 and the Oil Price Drop: The GCC Way.* PwC. https://www.strategyand.pwc.com/m1/en/covid-19-oil-price-drop-gcc.html

Talbot, V. (2020). *COVID-19 in MENA: Toward a Shift in the Regional Balance of Power in Dacrema, Eugenio ad Valeria Talbot eds, The MENA Region vs COVID-19: One Challenge, Common Strategies?* Mediterranean Dialogues, Italian Institute for International Political Studies. https://www.ispionline.it/sites/default/files/pubblicazioni/ispi_dossier_menavscovid19.pdf

Thucydides (1919). *History of the Peloponnesian War, Volume I: Books 1–2.* Loeb Classical Library. Cambridge, Harvard University Press.

UN (2020a). *The Impact of COVID-19 on the Arab Region an Opportunity to Build Back Better.* United Nations, New York, US. https://www.un.org/sites/un2.un.org/files/sg_policy_brief_covid- 19_and_arab_states_english_version_july_2020.pdf

UN (2020b). *The Impact of COVID-19 on the Arab Region an Opportunity to Build Back Better.* United Nations, New York, US. https://unsdg.un.org/sites/default/files/2020-07/sg_policy_brief_covid-19_and_arab_states_english_version_july_2020.pdf

Walt, S. M., & Belfer, R. (2020). *In the Post-Pandemic World, Big Brother Will Be Watching.* https://foreignpolicy.com/2020/05/16/future-government-powers-coronavirus-pandemic

World Bank. (2021). MENA Crisis Tracker – 12/13/2021. The World Bank. https://thedocs.worldbank.org/en/doc/0e069afd8d93a7a439f395e999772f88-0280032021/original/MENA-Crisis-Tracker-12-13-2021.pdf

World Bank (2022). *Global Economic Prospects: Middle East and North Africa.* World Bank. Washington, D.C. https://thedocs.worldbank.org/en/doc/cb15f-6d7442eadedf75bb95c4fdec1b3-0350012022/related/Global-Economic-Prospects-January-2022-Analysis-MENA.pdf

Wrage, A. (2020). *The Pandemic Will Be a Boon for Good Government.* https://foreignpolicy.com/2020/05/16/future-government-powers-coronavirus-pandemic

Index

Note: **Bold** page numbers refer to tables; *italic* page numbers refer to figures and page numbers followed by "n" denote endnotes.